Anatomia, 1838

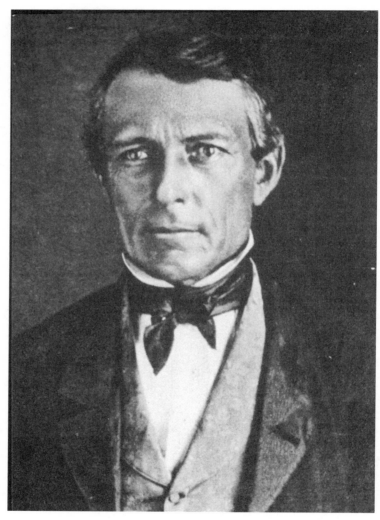

Gerrit P. Judd, M.D., 1803–1873

Anatomia, 1838

Gerrit P. Judd

Hawaiian Text
with English Translation
by
Esther T. Mookini

University of Hawai'i Press
Honolulu

This translation project was funded in part by the Division of Health Careers, Diversity and Development, Bureau of Health Professions, Health Resources Administration, Department of Health and Human Services.

This book is published with the support of Native Hawaiian Center of Excellence, John A. Burns School of Medicine.

The original text of Anatomia *was made available by the Hawai'i Medical Library.*

Printed in the United States of America

08 07 06 05 04 03   6 5 4 3 2 1

Library of Congress Cataloging-in-Publication Data

Judd, Gerrit Parmele, 1803–1873.
    [Anatomia. English & Hawaiian]
    Anatomia, 1838 / Gerrit P. Judd ; Hawaiian text with English translation by Esther T. Mookini.
    p. ; cm.
    Includes bibliographical references and index.
    English and Hawaiian.
    ISBN 0-8248-2585-3 (cloth : alk. paper)
    1. Human anatomy—Handbooks, manuals, etc. I. Mookini, Esther T. II. Title.
    [DNLM: 1. Anatomy. WZ 290 J92a 2003a]
    QM23 .J83 2003
    611—dc21

                                                        2002032107

Designed by Bookcomp, Inc.
Printed by The Maple-Vail Book Manufacturing Group

To the ten Hawaiian students who graduated from Hawaiʻi's first medical school, founded by Dr. Judd, in 1872: Daniel P. Aumai; Henry P. Kaili; Jno. Kalama; Geo. W. Kalopapela; Jno. W. Kalua; S.W. Kanealii, Jr.; S. K. Kauai, Jr.; Jno. Kelia; Henry Mana; and S. Naonohi.

To O. A. Bushnell, *kuu hoaloha.*

Finally, special thanks to Dr. Gerrit P. Judd, who throughout his life championed the cause of Hawaiian health and well-being, and left a vast legacy that is still with us today.

CONTENTS

FOREWORD

O. A. Bushnell

You who are well acquainted with schoolrooms are asked not to take lightly this little book, because it is a treasure from Hawai'i's history preserved for you since 1838 and presented to you now to regard in awe, as you learn anatomy from the bones of the human body and the tissues that hold them together.

When Protestant missionaries from New England reached Hawai'i in 1820, they were distressed to find that the islanders did not have a written language and therefore could not read the Holy Scriptures. So the missionaries listened to Hawaiians speaking among themselves and by 1824 devised a written language for them, consisting of twelve letters all borrowed from the English alphabet and "pronounced in the Italian manner." It helped reproduce the sounds of the rich Hawaiian vocabulary. Hawaiians eagerly attended the missionaries' many one-room schools to learn their new language. By 1850, Hawai'i became one of the few literate nations in the world. Thus, by this method of universal education resembling the American system Hawaiians entered the modern world.

Today, few of Hawai'i's residents remember to thank the missionaries for their great contributions to our education. In their schools, especially the first high school founded in 1831 at Lahainaluna on Maui, the missionaries taught Hawaiians something about the many arts and sciences that distinguish the great world beyond Hawai'i's shores. Graduates from the high school at Lahainaluna, sometimes called Mission Seminary, in their turn became teachers in smaller local schools.

Keeping Hawaiians alive after the arrival of Captain Cook's expedition in 1778 was difficult because they died faster than they managed to be born. Infectious disease brought in by visiting mariners killed many at appalling rates. Not a child born in all Hawai'i in 1843 lived more than two years. For the missionaries this mortality was a major concern. They tried by many means to slow the death rates. Among those means was a course in basic medicine taught by Dr. G. P. Judd, the only medical missionary, who remained for his entire life in the Kingdom of Hawai'i after his arrival in 1828.

To interest his students in the fundamentals of medicine, Judd resolved to write a textbook in anatomy. Learned though he was, he did not undertake the task without a mode. From Boston, the missionary headquarters in New England, he obtained a copy of *Class Book of Anatomy Designed for Schools*, written by Dr. Jerome V. C. Smith and published in 1834. Smith's text consisted of 290 pages and 110 engravings. Judd did not translate Dr. Smith's book directly; instead, he followed Smith's organization and prepared a text in the new written Hawaiian language, a small book of sixty pages with a separate section of fifty-eight engravings. These illustrations are remarkable in themselves; they were etched by students attending the Mission Seminary at Lahainaluna. Actually, they were copied from drawings made by Edward Bailey, a teacher who was stationed at the Mission Seminary, Lahainaluna, and later at the Female Seminary in Wailuku on Maui, and by Miss Persis Thurston, daughter of Reverend and Mrs. Asa Thurston of Kailua, Kona. The engravings were inscribed on copper plates provided by generous ships' captains who could spare

bits and pieces of larger plates intended to be used as sheathing on ships' bottoms as protection against ravages of sea
mollusks, which can bore holes in wooden hulls. The
engravings in *Anatomia* were assembled in a section by themselves, unlike those in Smith's book, which were interspersed
throughout his text. The names of three students at Lahinaluna who signed their works are known: Momona,
Kalama, and Kepohoni. According to Huc-Mazlet
Luquiens, a teacher of art at the University of Hawaiʻi in the
1930s, all the prints "display excellent draftsmanship, preci-
sion of techniques and understanding of the character of the
work."

Dr. Judd's *Anatomia* clearly shows his devotion to the edu-
cational and medical needs of the Hawaiian people. Think of
Dr. Judd. In spite of his many duties—as physician to all the
mission stations as well as to the native Hawaiians around
him, as adviser to chiefs, and as interpreter and translator for
the government—he somehow found the time to write a
textbook on a subject for which he had to create a new vocabulary and to explain medical functions and anatomical shapes
in words that a Hawaiian student was able to understand.
Think of the students at the Mission Seminary at
Lahainaluna, unaccustomed to chairs and desks, bent over
their etchings when they had never before handled a pen.
Imagine you yourself recently sent from your distant home
to attend the school at Lahinaluna, where almost everything
was new, different, and complicated, especially when you
were told to etch into pieces of copper things you had never
seen before, parts of the human body you could not have
seen until they were stripped of their coverings of flesh. (Possibly medical kahuna who separated the flesh of dead chiefs
from their bones helped in this process.)

Awesome is a term used too easily these days, too glibly,
yet it is the very word that describes Dr. Judd's *Anatomia*.
Think of the primitive conditions under which it was pro-

duced. Think of Dr. Judd in hot and humid Honolulu, dressed in the missionary's proper clothing—a flannel shirt, complete with a linen neck cloth, a woolen suit—leaning over the type font, carefully setting by hand the borrowed English letters, transforming them into newly minted Hawaiian phrases, then locking them into wooden frames that fit into the ancient mission press, then brushing ink over the new terms in order to obtain an imprint on a thin sheet of paper imported from Boston, six months' voyage away. Judd and his crew labored happily over those pages because they believed that they revealed the mechanisms that made and moved the Creator's most awesome creation—MAN.

PREFACE

Benjamin B. C. Young, M.D.

The background of *Anatomia* and the life of Dr. Gerrit Parmele Judd are described by Kiki Mookini in her introduction and by O. A. Bushnell in his foreword. Yet the purpose of the Native Hawaiian Center of Excellence (NHCOE) in republishing this book needs to be documented and thanks given to those who lent a hand in its publication.

The mission of NHCOE is to promote the health and wellness of all Native Hawaiians utilizing vehicles of research, leadership training, faculty development, curricula, and cultural competence, and expanding information resources to improve the knowledge base of Hawai'i's medical history. This fascination with Hawai'i's medical history led us to *Anatomia*. It is an important book because it is the only Western medical text published in the Hawaiian language describing anatomical landmarks. For example, the word *puna* is used to describe the matrix of bone held together like lime cement. It was at Honolulu harbor, Oahu, where Hawaiians would dive for the coral limestone used as mortar to join the huge coral blocks in the building of Kawaiahao Church. The clavicle is called *iwi lei* because a lei encircling the neck rested on this bone. One reclines on the humerus, the *iwi uluna* or the pillow bone, because the head rests on that bone like a pillow.

Anatomia is an elementary textbook, simple in descriptions and uncomplicated as a basic structural guide. Yet it was published at a time when some of the most important discoveries in Western medicine were not yet postulated. It would be another ten years before Ignaz Semmelweis determined that the washing of hands would prevent thousands of women from dying of childbirth fever. Twenty-five years after *Anatomia*, Louis Pasteur promulgated his germ theory.

Dr. Judd used Hawaiian words and descriptions that assist us today in appreciating the Hawai'i of the 1800s. He sermonizes frequently throughout the text. The religious admonitions make us constantly aware of his strict Calvinist background. We anticipate this work will be valued by linguists, historians, religious scholars, and cultural experts.

There are many to whom we owe much gratitude for assistance. The suggestion for doing this translation initially came from Dr. Iwalani Else, former recruitment coordinator for NHCOE. This project would never have come to pass had it not been for Kiki Mookini and her unflinching diligence and steady progress over two years. Medical historian Dr. O. A. Bushnell provided us with patient guidance along the way. Special thanks are extended to Barbara Dunn of the Hawaiian Historical Society and to Marilyn Reppun of the Hawaiian Mission Children's Society Library. To those who helped in reading the first drafts, Dr. Scott Lozanoff, chair of anatomy at JABSOM; Dr. Kathleen Durante, pediatrician; Dr. Scott Miles, cardiologist; Dr. Marjorie Mau, endocrinologist; Dr. Robert Simmons, orthopedic surgeon; internist Dr. Melvin Chang; pathologists Dr. Thomas Reppun and Dr. Ann Catts; attorney and physician Dr. R. Konane Mookini, and hematologist Dr. Kekuni Blaisdell, we convey our *mahalo pumehana*. The staff of Hawaii Medical Library, Director John Breinich and librarians Marilyn Ching and Leilani Marshall, were especially helpful. We are appreciative for Kathy Tanaka's (NHCOE secretary) patient and untiring support and assistance during the tedious meetings when she kept the minutes of our proceedings and dependably prepared draft copies for our review. It is always difficult to arrange the financial details of a publication, especially within an academic bureaucracy, and we thank Todd Nakamura, administrative officer of NHCOE for this task. We appreciate Nanette Purnell's relentless pressure at keeping us on schedule, especially during those periods of seemingly excruciating stagnation. Dr. Shannon Hirose-Wong, Dr. Martina Kamaka, Ms. Mele Look, and Mr. Kaloa Robinson provided many suggestions during our ongoing NHCOE meetings.

To Kaina Young, we owe much for his patient review of all the rough drafts, for serving as special assistant to Kiki Mookini, and for preparing the final format for submission.

To Masako Ikeda, who, with kind encouragement and diplomatic suggestions through every stage of the project, made us aware that even though she was born in Japan and raised in Malaysia and Singapore, she could teach all of us special meanings of the word *aloha*.

Finally, we could never adequately repay the love and dedication that Dr. Gerrit P. Judd showered upon the Hawaiians. In his lifetime, he saw the rapid decline of the *kanaka maoli* population. He helped to rescue the kingdom of Hawai'i from several foreign takeovers, especially in the tumultuous period of King Kamehameha III's reign. Records at the State of Hawai'i Archives describe his unstinting labors during the smallpox epidemic of 1853. He provided invaluable assistance in the training of the future kings, Kamehameha IV and Kamehameha V. Even during the waning years of his life, he still found the stamina to start Hawai'i's first medical school in 1870. Whenever a call came, his response was always like Isaiah of old, "Here am I . . . send me."

Although this book was written by Gerrit Parmele Judd, M.D., it would not be out of place for us to also have this English translation dedicated to him.

It would take very little time to drive *mauka* on Nuuanu Avenue to Oahu Cemetery and find Dr. Judd's final resting place. If one sits on the wall surrounding the family plot, one can hear the sounds of birds as they flutter among the headstones. The epitaph on Dr. Judd's marker is simple, "Hawaii's Friend." Over 130 years have passed since his death and he still remains Hawai'i's friend.

Anatomia will be a catalyst to help us produce future publications that will further link health and Hawaiian culture.

INTRODUCTION

Esther T. Mookini

Gerrit Parmele Judd, M.D., a medical missionary, graduated from Fairfield Medical College, Fairfield, New York, in 1825. He arrived in Honolulu in 1828, along with Rev. Lorrin Andrews and the Third Company of American Protestant missionaries sent by the American Board of Commissioners for Foreign Missions out of Boston (*Missionary Album*, 128). Before leaving for the Sandwich Islands mission, Judd and the others were given a Hawaiian language word list by Elisha Loomis, a member of the Pioneer Company that had arrived in Hawai'i in 1820. Five weeks before arriving in Hawai'i on March 30, 1828, Dr. Judd copied the Hawaiian words into a book of 128 pages (Judd IV, 96). Dr. Judd's arrival in Honolulu turned out to be timely because Dr. Abraham Blatchely, the only missionary physician, who came in 1823, had left the islands two years earlier. Dr. Judd, like Dr. Blatchely, not only attended to the medical needs of the missionaries but also to those of the native Hawaiians. In a matter of a few years, Judd developed his bilingual/bicultural talent as exhibited in *Anatomia*'s anatomical terms and functions explained in Hawaiian frames of reference. After being in the islands a few years, both Dr. and Mrs. Judd became fluent in the native tongue. In the 1830s, Dr. Judd was able to teach in the native schools and to preach in the native churches. In 1839, he reported to the mission that he had been occupied during the year as interpreter and translator for the government, an employment of much importance. On December 3, 1840, he was called "physician, interpreter, adviser and manager of the nation" (*Fragments, IV,* 97, 99).

In 1831, the first high school was established in Lahaina, Maui, by the American missionaries to train native school-teachers, theoretically and practically, the best methods of communicating instruction to others. In 1837, the name was changed from Lahainaluna High School to Mission Seminary. It was referred to as the seminary at Lahainaluna but most often called simply Lahainaluna (Kuykendall, v. 1, 111, 321, 364).

The school's only teacher during the first year was Rev. Lorrin Andrews, who not only prepared the school's curriculum by translating American textbooks into Hawaiian, but also built the schoolhouse with the help of the students. The main course of study was the Bible, for which the single-volume translation into Hawaiian began in 1827 and was completed in 1839 (Judd, A. F., 52–59).

Rev. Ephraim Clark, Rev. Sheldon Dibble, and a printer, Edmund Rogers, were sent to help Rev. Andrews, as more and more students were attending the seminary. In only three years the curriculum included geography, Greek, Hawaiian grammar and composition, geometry, trigonometry, arithmetic, and natural sciences. This same year, 1834, copper plate engraving was added to the curriculum (Lecker, 89–90). None of the missionaries knew the technique of copper plate engraving, and so Rev. Andrews decided to teach himself and the students the art. Spare pieces from large sheets of copper were obtained from ship masters. Copper plate sheathing from sailing ships was used from 1833 to 1843. During those ten years, 150 plates were engraved and printed at Lahainaluna, ranging in size from a wall map of the Hawaiian Islands, which used six plates, to Dr. Judd's *Anatomia* with fifty-eight engravings, using nineteen copper plates (Andrews, R. W., 13; *Missionary Album,* 129). Some of the engravers who signed their work were the students

Momona, Kalmua [Kalama], Nuyana [Nuuanu], Kapeau, and Kepohoni (van Patten, 2–3).

In ten years Judd's medical responsibility had increased so much that he wrote to the American Board requesting assistance. Whenever he could, he would enlist native Hawaiians as assistants. One such man was Hookano, his medical student, a graduate of Lahainalua, of whom Mrs. Judd said: "He was a valuable assistant both in the preparation of medicines and in prescribing for office patients" (Judd, L., 128).

Dr. Judd was especially concerned about the Hawaiian people, who were so susceptible to introduced diseases and who had little knowledge of Western-style hygiene. He wrote: "The state of the natives cries loudly for help. They are fast decreasing in numbers" (Judd IV, 87). He devoted much time to educating the missionaries in outlying stations so that they could administer simple medical aid to each other and to their Hawaiian congregations. He wrote to the American Board of Commissioners for Foreign Missions to send medical books to all the mission stations, saying, "Every station must be supplied with medicines for the use of both missionaries and people and the need for books is obvious in order to guide those who administer them." For the immediate use of missionaries and natives alike he prepared a handwritten treatment book in the Hawaiian language, which was later translated into English (ibid., 90–91). The first edition of Dr. Jerome V. C. Smith's *Class Book of Anatomy Designed for Schools* (1834) may have been sent to Dr. Judd in answer to his request for medical books.

In 1835, the American Board ordered Dr. Judd to prepare a textbook on anatomy for the students at the seminary. The following year, 1836, of the eighty-four students at Lahainaluna, one was sent to Judd in Honolulu to assist him in his medical work (Lecker, 145). That same year Rev. Andrews published, at the Lahainaluna Press, his *Vocabulary of the Hawaiian Language*, which was greatly expanded in 1865 and retitled *Dictionary of the Hawaiian Language*. Rev. Andrews credited Dr. Judd for the Hawaiian names of the bones, muscles, and ligaments of the human system (L. Andrews, 3).

The following year, 1837, the missionaries asked the American Board to appoint and send a medical man as a teacher of chemistry, mineralogy, botany, and medicine to Lahainaluna. Rev. Ephraim Clark at the Mission Seminary (Lahainaluna) wrote: "The Seminary is needed to raise up medical practitioners. It has been ascertained that the inhabitants of the islands are on the decrease. The causes of this are various but the neglect of the sick and improper medical treatment hold a prominent place. A large proportion of infants die within a year after birth, owing to neglect or improper treatment. The sick are often hurried into eternity by the absurd practice of superstitious doctors. It is hoped that young men will be brought forward in the Mission Seminary who may become skilled in the healing art and in this way supplant the quackery of the present native doctors and thus contribute to save the nation from extinction. A small work has been prepared by Dr. Judd as he is now (July 1837) engaged in teaching a class in the Seminary this branch of medical science" (Clark, 349).

At the general meeting in Honolulu, June 1838, it was reported that *Anatomia* was finished in that year, June 1837–June 1838 (personal communication, Marilyn Reppun, librarian, Hawaiian Mission Children's Society Library). In March 1838, Dr. Judd's neighbor, Amos Cooke, noted in his journal: "Yesterday . . . called at bro. Dimond's, also on Dr. Judd. . . . Dr. showed us some engravings of a Lahainaluna engraver—very well done for a native. The Dr. is preparing a book on anatomy in native" (*Hawaiian National Bibliography*, v. 1, 174–175). Dr. Judd lectured on medical topics and was invited by the Lahaina mission in 1837–1838 to give annual medical lectures at Lahainaluna Seminary but this project never materialized (*Fragments*, II, 106–107).

In 1838, the American Board answered Judd's appeal for a teacher saying, "To hire such a teacher would have to wait for more prosperous time and for them to have patience and that perhaps such a medical teacher could be sent to Lahainaluna but not at this time" (Lecker, 161). That year the Mission Press in Honolulu published Dr. Judd's *Anatomia*. Although the printing records show that 500 copies were printed, letters from Rev. Andrews to Dr. Judd (private communication) indicate that only about 200 copies had the engraved plates inserted. The minutes of the 1838 Delegate Meeting record an edition of 200 copies. Dr. Judd prepared the text in Honolulu and an order was placed for the appropriate stereotype plates from Boston. For some reason these did not arrive, and Dr. Judd arranged to have them manufactured in Lahainaluna (*Hawaiian National Bibliography*, v. 1, 175). The Lahainaluna students copied and engraved fifty-eight of Smith's 110 engravings. Their skill was said to have been remarkable (van Patten, 2). Dr. Judd used Smith's 280-page *Class Book of Anatomy Designed for Schools* as the basis for his own book on anatomy, but clearly the sixty-page *Anatomia* was not a direct translation of Dr. Smith's 280-page book. Dr. Judd's explanation and descriptions of the parts of the body and functions of different organs and muscles were in his own words and especially designed for the Hawaiian students at Lahainaluna. He used examples of things Hawaiian so that the students would be able to understand anatomy. Throughout *Anatomia* Dr. Judd lectured on the proper care of the body.

In 1839, the members of the Hawaiian Evangelical Association met and adopted the report of its Committee on Medical Instruction, which said: "There is and has been a greater need of native doctors than of native lawyers. The missionaries have educated the native pastors. The native lawyers have educated themselves . . . but the medical profession has been like a sealed book" (Bushnell, 396).

Finally, after thirty-two years, in 1870 the legislators appropriated $4,000 to the Bureau of Public Instruction "for the medical education of Hawaiian Youth," and appointed Dr. Judd to take charge of the instruction of these young men. On November 9, 1870, he opened a school with ten pupils. Certainly in Dr. Judd the kingdom had acquired a physician of great ability, possibly the islands' most experienced physician, and a teacher dedicated to his missionary's goal of bringing both physical and spiritual succor to the Hawaiian people" (Bushnell, 396, 400).

Anatomia was published in 1838. The diacritical marks that are being used today were not in use in the nineteenth century when the missionaries put the Hawaiian language into print. According to Al Schutz, the missionaries did use glottal stops but only for a few words. Since Dr. Judd's *Anatomia* had no diacriticals, I have chosen to maintain the Hawaiian language as it appeared in the original text. In the entire textbook I found some typos and mistakes, which I have so noted in the annotations. The reader in the Hawaiian language is strongly advised to use the 1865 *Dictionary of the Hawaiian Language* by Rev. Lorrin Andrews. This translation with its mistakes is my responsibility.

My gratitude goes to the Native Hawaiian Center of Excellence for their development of this project. The following are in my *lei aloha* for their time and help: Jason Achiu, Dr. Kekuni Blaisdell, Dr. Ann Catts, Dr. Melvin Chang, Dr. Kathleen Durante, Dr. David Fong, Frances Frazier, Dr. Martina Kamaka, Judy Kearney, Patrick Kehoe, Laurie Kuribayashi, Esq., Gerald Langley, Lani Maa Lapilio, Esq., Jodie Mattos, Dr. Darlene Fong Metter, Dr. R. Konane Mookini, Dr. Thomas Reppun, Marilyn Reppun, James Rumford, Albert Schutz, Susan Shaner, Dr. Robert Simmons, Kaina Young.

Anatomia
A Translation

This is a book that explains the nature
of the human body.

Written in the Hawaiian language in order
to teach the students of the high school
at Lahainaluna.

Oahu: Mission Press, 1838.

ANATOMY

3   This word, *anatomy*, means the nature of the body and all the
things placed in it: the bones, muscles, ligaments, *olona*,[1]
joints, blood vessels, *aa*,[2] protuberances, intestines, and fluids. All these things and what they do inside the body to benefit man will be explained in this book.

From ancient times in enlightened countries, many people pursued the study of anatomy. They looked carefully at
bones. They cut open a large number of corpses, carefully
examined the intestines so as to know the nature of everything that the eyes saw. Much of it is understood at the present time. And so, enlightened people practiced the wisdom
of God, the one who made and indeed put and kept in order
the extraordinary things in their bodies. The ungodly cannot say "there is no God" because they witnessed him
through his great work. Here is another excellent thing that
came from their research: they discovered the nature of diseases and pain. They knew medicines. The experts of medicines today are very skillful, not like those of the past. Jesus
and the miracle workers, helped by God, were the only ones
most skilled in administering medicine.

REGARDING BONES

The responsibility of bones in the body is great. They are firm, *maloeloe*,[3] and are hard, *oolea*.[4] If man was made without bones, such as the sea cucumber, *loli*,[5] then how could he possibly stand up? How could he move about? How indeed could he labor? Some bones protect—for example, the head bones protect the brain and the ribs protect the lungs. Most of the bones are levers, *une*,[6] such as a stick used to move a heavy object. Bones do the same and it is the muscles that pull.

4   During childhood, the bones are soft and flexible so they are not quick to break. When a man is full grown, they are hard, and when he is an old man, they break frequently because they are dry. Lime [calcium], *puna*,[7] is the thing that hardens bones. When a bone is burned in fire, then lime is clearly seen. It is white but not exactly like true calcium because several things are mixed in it. Cartilage, *pilali*,[8] is another thing inside bones. It is a very important foundation for bones. To explain cartilage, take the thigh bone of a chicken and put it into some acid mixed with water. Let this stand for perhaps three nights. Then the calcium will have been eaten up by the acid. The hardness of the bone is gone. It is soft, clear, and transparent, almost like glass.

During pregnancy, the child's bones are only cartilage. Later on, blood brings calcium and deposits it in the center of the cartilage. It is getting ready for that child to grow, changing soft bones into hard bones because calcium had entered inside the cartilage. Look inside a long bone and you will see a hole for blood to enter.

This work begins in the very center of the bone. If it is a large bone, it starts at the sides and calcium goes into the center of the cartilage, looking like grains of wood, *nao*,[9] joining one to another. If it is a long bone, calcium is deposited in the center and also in the heads. This calcium is not mixed until the person is an adult, so until then [the earthy portions of] long bones will crumble, *helelei*,[10] and the waste [dried-up portions, *maloo*],[11] will be [removed and] renewed. (See Smith, 38.)

If a bone breaks, the places that broke are joined together again, then blood will bring and deposit calcium surrounding the [broken] places. That is the thing that joins the bone again until [the bone is] firm.

Some bones are flat, some are long and round, and others are irregular. They are completely covered with something gauzelike and smooth, which is the wrapping of the bone. This is what takes away the roughness as the bones slip and slide, moving between the muscles.

The large long bones are hollow, *hakahaka*,[12] but firm and do not break suddenly. They are light in weight and it is here that fat is stored. Here perhaps is the responsibility of fat in 5   bones. When a person is sick, he will not be able to eat. It is not good for his stomach to have food in it just to be filled since food will turn into something bitter and hot and there will be gnawing in his stomach. It is then that the aforementioned fat will be sent for and taken to all parts of the body through the blood. It is the thing that strengthens a person when he is sick. But if the sickness takes a long time, that fat will be spent; then the fat from the entire body is brought in and the loss of weight of that sick person will be over quickly. When the sickness is over and food is in the stomach again, strengthening the body, then the aforementioned fat which was brought in earlier returns and the bones are filled again with fat. Because of these things it is necessary to put aside food during the time of sickness because the stomach will be nauseated by the food since it knows food is a burden. Don't be afraid if the sick person sinks down with weakness for want of food. If the stomach refuses food, the person will not die immediately of hunger. How great is God's generosity because he made preparations of fat inside bones in order to sustain the body at the time of sickness.

There are 240 bones in our bodies. In order to learn them they are divided into three divisions. 1. The bones of the head. 2. The bones of the body itself. 3. The bones of the limbs [extremities].

THE BONES OF THE HEAD

The head has 63 bones:

8 bones of the head itself [skull], which surround the brain
14 bones of the face
32 teeth (of an adult)
 8 bones of the ears
 <u>1</u> bone of the tongue
63

Heads of people are not at all alike when looking at them. God made slight differences one from another. The same is true of faces. In searching through countries, no two people have the same face. Some twins' faces are almost alike. But if you look carefully, then their differences will be seen.

6

It is very important in unenlightened countries to change the natural shape of the heads of their children into new shapes. Some squeeze the sides of the head to flatten the sides. For other people it is the forehead. The people of Hawaii believe that a handsome head is a head flattened at the forehead and the back of the head. In enlightened countries they just leave the heads of their children alone because it was by the grace of God that made them.

BONES OF THE HEAD

1 forehead bone, *iwi lae*,[13] at the forehead. Os frontis, frontal.

2 side (*hua*) bones, *iwi hua*,[14] at the sides of the head. Ossa parietalia, parietal.

1 rear bone, *iwi hope*,[15] at the back of the head. Os occipitis, occipital.

2 temple bones, *iwi maha*,[16] at the temples. Ossa temporum, temporal.

1 sieve bone, *iwi kanana*,[17] between the brain and the base of the nose. Os ethmoides, ethmoid.

1 bat bone, *iwi opeapea*,[18] inside and under the brain. Os sphenoides, sphenoid.

FOREHEAD, OR FRONTAL BONE

This is a single bone when a person is an adult, but when a child is born it is divided in two, in the middle. It goes from top downward, becoming two bones. It is a thin bone whose features are like that of an oyster, *olepe*.[19] There is a place full of holes at the apex joining with the nose bones between the two sides of the forehead bone, at the inside and the outside. This is the thing that makes the voice resound. Because of the empty space, the sound is like that of a drum, *pahu*.[20] When one gets sick, he has what is called a stopped-up nose. The hole through which the wind enters into the aforesaid empty space is closed; hence the voice is heavy sounding. At this bone there is a part of the eyeball socket and on the side there is a flat side or ridge for the adhering of the temporal muscle, which pulls the upper jaw bone. Also at this bone are edges, places where the eyebrows join.

WALL, OR PARIETAL BONES

These bones are flat but not truly flat. On the outside they swell out [convex], and on the inside they fall in [concave].

7   The parietal bones come to the center of the skull and they resemble a square. It is the large bone of the head and is frequently broken in battle, *kaua.*[21]

BACK, OR OCCIPITAL BONE

This bone is very thick because many muscles are attached to it which pull the head up. It has a long part underneath where it is joined with the bat or sphenoid bone. There is a hole in the underside, a very large hole, perhaps one inch in diameter. It is from here that the spinal marrow goes down into the spine and branches out to the entire body. At the edge of the large hole are four small holes, and it is here that the head joins with the first bone of the spine. At the hole near the adjoining bone is where the nerve of the tongue emerges. It is the taste nerve, *aalolo hoao.*[22]

TEMPLE, OR TEMPORAL BONE

This bone is surrounded by the frontal bone, the parietal bone, the occipital bone, and the sphenoid bone. This is an irregularly shaped bone. The thin, flat side is called partly scaly, *unahi,*[23] [squamous part], the thick side is called partly hard, *oolea,*[24] [petrous part]. It is here that the hearing things, the ears, are. It has a projection that is joined to the band of the cheek [malar] bone in front of the ear, and there is a protuberance behind the ear called the base of the ear. This bone has a long thing on the underside. It is perhaps one and a half inches long, looking like a needle, *kui,*[25] and so it is called the styloid process. There are many muscles for swallowing, which are attached to the styloid process of the temporal bone.

This bone has many holes. There is the external ear hole.

It is a large hole and surrounded by bony edges. The ear is here. An internal ear hole is a large hole in the back side of the petrous part of the bone. The hearing [auditory] nerve of the ear enters through this hole. There is a small hole at the base of the ear for a nerve going to the cheek. There is an irregularly shaped hole where sounds from the mouth go into the ear. There is a cavity in this bone where the lower jaw is joined. Here is another: look inside and you will see irregularly shaped openings adhering to the brain with space for the artery for the wrapping of the brain.

8

SIEVE, OR ETHMOID BONE

This name is given for the many tiny holes pierced in this bone, [making it appear] like a pepper shaker or a sieve. It is situated just below in the middle of the head under the brain at the base of the nose and also between the eyes. Should the bones of the head split apart and separate, then the ethmoid bone will be seen. There is a nerve that is branched out. The branches are numerous and are like white thread but short. They enter into the holes of this bone and it is here that they go into the nose. Its name is the smelling [olfactory] nerve and it is the thing that recognizes fragrant things it smells.

This [bone] is full of open spaces, light in weight, full of holes, in order for the voice to sound and to recognize a scent. It has a loose attachment, *lepe*,[26] like a cock's comb, standing in the center of the brain, and it is here that the partition of the brain is fixed. This bone has two smooth places, which are for the eye sockets. There is a partition in between that stands directly at the ridge of the nose. There are two rolled-up bones, each adhering to the sides of this partition, and it is here that the disease known as polypus, *iokupu*,[27] begins.

BAT, OR SPHENOID BONE

This bone closes the space [at the base] of the skull. If it is taken out and separated, it looks like a bat, hence its name. This bone adheres to fourteen other bones. The places called wings are at the temples, the small wings are a little inside. The feet are at the mouth where the upper teeth end. There are four feet, two inside and two outside. The eye socket side is inside the outer side of the eye socket. At the center of this bone there are four sharp points, almost like the upright posts of a bed, which are called corner posts. In the middle of these posts is a low place called the saddle.

9   There are two round holes under the front corner posts that are called the seeing [optic] holes because it is here that the optic nerves emerge and go into the eyes. Just a little behind are the large holes called the spread-out holes, where four nerves emerge at these holes and go into the eye-rolling muscles. In back are round holes, called long round holes. It is here that the nerve for the lower jaw bone emerges.

REGARDING THE JOININGS [SUTURES]
OF THE HEAD BONES

When a child is born, all the head bones are small and are not properly attached one to another. The head remains that way until the infant emerges from his cramped place. The head is soft at this time. The way out is very difficult and the pangs of childbirth are very strong. Then a bone overlaps, *lele*,[28] another; the head is lengthened out; it is very long and narrow. Here the grace of God is evident because if the bones at this time were joined together and the head was very hard, then birth could never occur. The child would die as well as his mother. The edges of the head bones of the child are yet to be finished. The space yet to be completed is called the fontanel. When the child is big, all the bones will have grown and will have correctly joined, one with another, in order to protect the brain from injury. However, places to be joined will not have all disappeared. A bone enters into another like hinged bones but it can get loose and separate. The joining of the bones is called the union of things sewn [suture]. If the head were left alone, its softness would be like it was at birth, and that is not good. Should a person fall down hard on his head, his brain might be badly injured and he could quickly die. We must not forget the love of the one who mercifully created this.

Regarding these things, we know about the foolishness of some people regarding their desire to enlarge the size of the fontanel. They would squeeze milk or place medicine on it to break it open. Yet they cannot break it apart. It is never the nature of milk to break the head open.

10   Here is another foolish thing: they would just leave the fontanel alone, not to be washed with water until dirt and filth were gone. They would plaster a rag on it and it would remain that way. Don't be afraid of washing the fontanel. Don't be afraid to touch it with your hand because if it is wrong to do so, why would you want to split it wide open? The head of a child is soft, so you must not hit his head hard with your hand. You must not hit or strike it, but a washrag is painless, and so use warm water and soap every day.

THE JOININGS [SUTURES]
OF THE HEAD

Four joinings [sutures] of the head, two fontanels.

1. Fontanel joining, *hoai manawa*,[29] [coronal suture], goes from one temple rising over to the top of the skull at one fontanel and descending to the other temple. This is the thing that joins the frontal and parietal bones.

2. Ridge of the house joining, *hoai kaupaku*,[30] [sagittal suture]. This is at the very top of the head, from the front or anterior fontanel to the back or posterior fontanel. Here the two parietal bones join and it looks like the ridge of a house.

3. The *L* joining, *hoai kala*,[31] [lambdoidal suture]. It is here in the back where the occipital and parietal bones join, from the base of the ear, rising up to the posterior fontanel and descending to the base of the other ear.

4. Temple joining, *hoai maha* [temporal suture]. This is the joining of the temporal, parietal, and frontal bones. The temporal bone rises above these bones like scales that cling to fish. That is the way it adheres.

1. The forward [anterior] fontanel is at the outside corners where the parietal bones join with the frontal bone.

2. The rear [posterior] fontanel is at the outside corners where the parietal bones join with the occipital bone. This is small. The anterior fontanel is large.

BONES OF THE FACE

2 upper jaw bones [maxilla]. They adhere to each other as one. Ossa maxillaria superiora.

2 cheek bones [malar]. At the cheeks. Ossa malarum.

2 nasal bones. Above the nose. Ossa nasi.

2 tear bones [lachrymal]. Inside the eye socket. Ossa lachrymalia.

2 roof-of-the-mouth bones [palate]. At the end of the upper jaw inside the mouth. Ossa palatina.

2 rolled-up-like-parchment bones [turbinated], *iwi owili*,[32] Inside the nose. Ossa turbinata.

11   1 partition bone [vomer], *iwi paku*.[33] In the center of the nose.

1 lower jaw bone [mandible]. Os maxillare inferius.

UPPER JAW BONES, OR MAXILLA

These bones are joined to one of the head bones and adhere one to the other so that there is little or no shaking when eating. The upper teeth have been put into the edge of this bone. It has a protuberance above the corners of the mouth and underneath the cheek bone. It is hollow inside and its name is the cave [antrum]. This hollow is where the voice sounds, in the same way as does the frontal bone. A side of this bone enters the eye socket, the side under and inside. A sharp projection rises at the nose as the threshhold for the nasal bones and it is here that it adheres to the frontal bone. This bone has a large hole inside the eye socket that goes on to the nose. There, tears flow and go all the way into the nose. There are two very small holes in the tear ducts, *luauhane*.[34] One is at the upper edge, the other at the lower edge. These are the holes where tears enter, but should a person cry very much, all the water cannot enter because the holes have no room, so then tears fall out all over the cheeks.

CHEEK, OR MALAR BONES

These bones are in front of the ears, joined with the temporal, maxilla, and frontal bones. Joining with the temporal bone is the band for the temple muscle and the chewing muscle that pulls the lower jaw up.

NOSE, OR NASAL BONES

These bones are an inch long, joined with the frontal bone. They adhere to each other. They lie directly over the nose like the board in front of a canoe, *kuapoi*.[35]

TEAR, OR LACHRYMAL BONES

These are very small bones. Their shapes are like that of fingernails in size and in thinness. They are inside the eye socket, *luamaka*,[36] on one side of the tear hole. If that aforementioned hole is blocked, skilled people have always pierced this bone for tears to flow.

12

ROOF OF THE MOUTH, OR PALATE BONES

These are two bones that are joined together. They are where the upper jaw bone ends at the palate. These bones were made as a partition between the mouth and the nose. These bones, the turbinated bones, and the nasal bones are the ones frequently destroyed by syphilis. It is the sickness that God gave as punishment to adulterous people.

ROLLED-UP BONES, OR TURBINATED BONES

Two of them are very far inside the nose, and it is here that the disease of the nose, polypus, grows. The bones are light in weight and thin and are rolled up like small rolls of parchment. The smelling [olfactory] nerves branch out and come out of the ethmoid bone and are spread out over the turbinated bones like a spider's web. This bone is small in the nose of a man, perhaps one inch long, but in a dog's nose and in other animals' noses it is very large. Thus perhaps due to the length of their noses, they are skillful in smelling for their food and in tracking down things they are searching for.

PARTITION BONE, OR VOMER

This is a single bone standing in the middle of the nose inside the post. The partition cartilage adheres to it and is joined with the upper jaw bone. Sometimes it stands to one side, not directly in the center of the nose.

LOWER JAW BONE, OR MANDIBLE

This bone is joined with the temple bones, a little below the band where there is a hinge in front of the ear. This bone has two branches where they join: one is called the hinge branch; the other, in front of it, is called the front branch. There is a small hole inside this bone, going from one side of the chin to the other side, where a vein and a nerve flow and branch out to the teeth.

CONCERNING TEETH

13   There are 32 teeth in an adult: 16 in the upper jaw and 16 in the lower jaw. Here are their names:

8 milk-eating teeth [incisors], *niho ai waiu*[37]
4 eye teeth [cuspids]
8 double teeth [bicuspids]
8 large double teeth [molars]
4 adult [wisdom teeth] *niho oo*[38]

The tooth is like a real bone, hard on the outside so that it can properly chew tough, *uaua*,[39] things. When a child is born, the teeth are in their places inside the jaw bones. The first teeth [baby or milk teeth], which will fall out, are on top and the fixed [permanent] teeth are underneath. When the child grows to perhaps six months old, a tooth will appear just like a planted seed sprouting out of the soil, *kupu*,[40] giving fruit. It takes two years for the first teeth, twenty of them, to grow. In perhaps the sixth year, a tooth will fall out and a new tooth will grow to fill up the space. It takes eighteen to perhaps twenty years for the wisdom teeth to grow. Thus they are called adult teeth, teeth of wisdom.

Some people are mistaken in saying that teeth are rooted at the base of the ears. That is not so. These teeth cannot crawl inside the jaw bone until they come to their places to emerge.

Let us remember God's goodness when he gave milk [to the mother] for the infant when he was born, and when the right time came for him to eat [solid] food he gave *hoawi*,[41] him teeth to chew.

Here is another thought: those people who think of withholding milk and feeding the child other things are foolish. It is not right to wean a child and feed him fish and poi when he has no teeth. He would die and yet death would not be quick, *wawae*,[42] because his stomach would not be able to keep all of these things down and so he would pine away, shrivel up, have sudden internal pains, get hot, have thrush perhaps, and diarrhea. Stop giving him solid food until he has teeth, which will come. Then the stomach will be ready, and fish and poi will become the things that will make the child strong and grow big.

14   Here is another [thought]. Do not just knock out and remove teeth. Leave them alone quietly just where they were planted by God. But if there is pain and perhaps the tooth is shaking, then remove it.

TONGUE BONE, OR HYOID

This is a single bone in the middle of the muscles of the tongue, above the round protuberance [laryngeal prominence, "Adam's apple"]. Its appearance is like that of the lower jaw but small and round, nearly like the size of a dollar.

BONES OF THE EAR

There are eight of these bones, four in one ear and four in the other. They are very small.

Hammer [malleus] bone, believed to look like a hammer.

Back [anvil, incus] bone, *iwi kua*,[43] for the anvil of a blacksmith [*amara*[44]].

Round bone, a very small bone. The mustard seed is large.

Stirrup, stapes, *keehi*,[45] bone looking like stirrups on a small saddle, *noho lio*.[46]

When things vibrate at the partition inside the ear, the long handle of the hammer bone [malleus] is pulled, its head comes down at a low place of the back bone [anvil], the tip of the back bone rises at the round bone, the stirrup is pulled, and there is a great shaking where the hearing [acoustic] nerve is flattened out. Our hearing is a wonderful thing, a mystery, and most difficult to explain clearly in the Hawaiian language.[47] If you want to see the ear bones, look for a head of a dog or perhaps a cow and look carefully inside the ear. A dry head bone is best, but if it is repeatedly thrown about, here and there and everywhere, then the bones will be destroyed. If such a bone is found, you will see that they are like those of a man.

BONES OF THE BODY

There are 53 bones named in the body:

24 spine bones [vertebrae]
24 side bones [ribs]
 1 chest bone [sternum]
 4 bones of the loins, *iwi ka*[48] [pelvis]
--
53

15   These fifty-three bones are the foundation upon which the limbs and the things that protect soft things [organs] are attached. Should they not be protected from hard objects, pain is quick to come. Within the spine is the extension of the brain that is called the spinal nerve [cord]. Within the chest are the liver and the heart. Within the region of the loins are the urinary bladder and the womb, *puuao.*[49]

BONES OF THE SPINE, OR VERTEBRAE

There are twenty-four of them: seven neck [cervical], twelve back [dorsal], and five loin [pelvic]. They are all firmly joined one to another. If you take the spine and look at it carefully, you will see three projections, two on the back side and one in the center. There are four places where they join together with another bone, two above and two below. The body of the bone is a bit round. Look at the big hole for the spinal nerve which goes down and branches in the middle of every second bone. It goes that way from top to bottom. The projections are for the attaching of muscles and ligaments to pull the body to stand upright and for the body to straighten up again after bending down. There is a tough cartilage in the middle of the bones adhering also to the bone. It allows the spine to bend a little or it will break.

If the height of a man is measured in the morning and he works hard that whole day and he is measured again, it will be plain to see that his height was shortened by perhaps one inch. Here is the thing that shortened him: standing upright with the muscles pulling hard will press down on the hard things [intervertebral disks], making them somewhat thin, and the spine will be shortened.

The first bone of the neck [atlas] is joined with the head. It is a joint for nodding the head. It is grooved and a projection of the second of the bones enters into the groove, like a

house post goes into the rafter.[50] Between the two the head
rolls back and forth and turns to look about.

SIDE BONES, OR RIBS

There are twenty-four of these bones, twelve on one side and
twelve on the other. Men and women have the same number. A head is joined to the back bone of the spine and in that
way there are twelve back bones. Another head is joined at
the chest bone [sternum]. This head is sticky in order to ease
proper breathing. The seven bones on top directly adhere
with the chest bone [sternum]. The last two bones are short
and merely float inside the muscles.

When a man inhales, the lungs fill up, the ribs rise up, and
then he exhales and the ribs go back down. In that way the
chest opens and shuts continually all day and night until life
ends.

CHEST BONE, OR STERNUM

This is a lightweight bone, one and a quarter inches wide, ten
inches long, sometimes. Where it is joined with the necklace
bone [clavicle] is its breadth. On the underside at the chest is
a cartilage. There are perhaps five bones of the chest during
childhood. When a person is an adult, the bones perhaps join
to become three and then at another time to only one.

CONCERNING THE BONES
OF THE LOINS, OR PELVIS

This is the full name of the four separate bones that are
joined, and because of the roundness they resemble a gourd,
ipu.[51] These bones are immovable; they are indeed the foundation upon which the body, the head, and the upper limbs sit.

2 hip bones, *iwi papakole*.[52] [Ossa innominata].

1 hollow of the back between the hip bones, *iwi kikala*.[53] [Sacrum]. Os sacrum.

1 anus bone, *iwi okole*.[54] [Os coccyx].

HIP BONES

These are two irregularly shaped bones. They are joined in the front, and in the back, they join with the hollow of the back bone, but the two are separated, *puanauweia*,[55] into three bones. The flattened-out bone at the hips is called the hip bones. Where the two join in the front is the pubic bone, *iwi puukole*,[56] and the place where a person sits down in a chair is called the buttocks bone, *iwi lemu*.[57] These bones are separated in childhood; when a person is an adult the three bones are joined to become one. They join in the cavity of the chicken egg, *hua moa*,[58] of the twist string on the thigh bone, *iwi hilo*[59] [femur]. Two-fifths of this cavity is for the hip bones, two-fifths for the buttocks bone, and one-fifth for the pubic bone. There is a rough border above the hip bone where muscles adhere greatly and it is called the border. Where the border ends in the front, there are two protuberances; the one above is called *kapai*,[60] the upper projection, and the one below is called the lower projection of the hip bone. There, between the buttocks bone and the pubic bone, is a large hole called a long circular hole. Where these bones join, one place is called the branch of the pubic bone and, another place, the branch of the buttocks bone. The hips of a woman spread out, a man's do not.

17

HOLLOW OF THE BACK BETWEEN THE HIP BONES, OR SACRUM

It is almost like a triangle: two sides are equal and the point of the joining is turned downward. This is a single bone, but in childhood there may be perhaps five. There are many holes within it, perhaps ten, where the branches of the spinal nerve emerge.

ANUS BONE, OR COCCYX

This adheres to the pointed place of the hip bone and is bent inward. Man may have one or two of this bone, but animals have a multitude called a tail.

BONES OF THE LIMBS

There are sixty-four bones of the upper limbs and sixty in the lower limbs. They are double; one side of the body is the same as the other side.

BONES OF THE UPPER LIMBS, OR UPPER EXTREMETIES

2 paddle bones, *iwi hoehoe*[61] [scapula]	Shoulder bones
2 necklace bones, *iwi lei*[62] [clavicle]	
2 pillow bones, *iwi uluna*[63] [humerus]	
2 cubit bones, *iwi kubita*[64] [ulna]	
2 handle bones, *iwi kano*[65] [radius]	Long bones
16 hand protuberance bones, *iwi pulima*[66] [carpus]	
10 fan-shaped hand bones, *iwi peahi lima*[67] [metacarpus]	Small and round bones
23 hand branches, *iwi manamanalima*[68] [phalanges]	
___	
64	

18   ## PADDLE BONES, OR SCAPULA

This is a spread-out, thin bone shaped like a triangle, floating in between the muscles of the shoulders, not attached
to any bone, except to the necklace bone [clavicle]. This
bone has two projections: the flat projection where it is
joined with the clavicle and a ridge where it goes as far as
the width of that bone. The noselike projection, on the
inside, is a protection for the pillow bone [humerus]. Without this it would slip down inside. The flat projection pro-
tects from above. In between these projections there is a
small cavity for the head of the pillow bone [humerus],
where this bone rotates.

NECKLACE BONE, OR CLAVICLE

It lies horizontally between the sternum and the scapula at
the shoulders. It is the thing that secures the shoulder joint.
The important function of the clavicle is to brace the shoulders from falling forward and downward. If this bone should
break, then the shoulders would quickly fall down. There is
a large artery under the clavicle.

PILLOW BONE, OR HUMERUS

This bone is long and straight and has a round head on top
where it is joined with the scapula. It is a little spread out at
the tip below where it enters the cubit bone [ulna], [at the
elbow]. This protuberance is a true hinge, it never rotates
like the shoulder. It folds over on top and is straightened out
below. That is the extent of its movement.

The bone joints can rotate properly as they have heads and
cavities to rotate in. These joints are called floating joints;

but if the rotating cannot be done, and all they can do is bend away from and bend toward, then they are called hinge joints. The humerus has a floating joint at the shoulders and a hinged joint at the elbow.

There is a space above this bone for the tendon of a muscle called the sweet potato, *uala* [biceps].[69] It is the thing that bends the arm. There are protuberances on each side of the aforementioned space where the muscles secure the rotating of the arm. There is a long ridge or flat side in the middle only for the muscles. At the flat extension beneath, there are the outside protuberance and the inside protuberance. Examine carefully the joining with the cubit bone [ulna] at the cavity where a joint enters. There is a small cavity in front of the first protuberance of the cubit bone [ulna]. Look also at the place where it joins together with the handle bone [radius]. Two long bones remain to be explained in the arm. They lie in the same way, attached to the heads, and they are equal in size.

19

CUBIT BONE, OR ULNA

Cubit is the name of this bone because it was the unit of measurement used by the ancient people when they measured a cubit. One cubit is measured from the elbow as far as the protuberance where this bone joins the wrist. Some people lengthen the cubit to the tip of the longest finger of the hand. The tip of this bone adheres to the pillow bone [humerus] and its appearance is like that of a whale bone, *iwi palaoa*.[70] The tongue [of the pendant] is the joint and the chest [of the pendant] is where the bone is secured or else it would slip forward and downward. This is called the front protuberance of the cubit bone [ulna]. The small head of this bone is attached to the handle bone [radius] and perhaps in a small way with the wrist bones.

HANDLE BONE, OR RADIUS

The small head of the radius adheres to the side of the ulna at the elbow just as the ulna adheres to the radius at the wrist. When the arm moves, a head rolls, then another head rolls, and the bones are turned against the hand at the radius. The hand is at the radius, which turn together in movement. The eight bones [in the wrist] are able to do so. This is not good because there are twelve bones there [radius, ulna, and two heads].

CONCERNING THE WRIST, OR CARPUS

There are eight irregularly shaped bones inside the wrist, with a sticky substance looking perhaps like crooked stones, built up on each other, embedded solidly in mortar, *uahau, uhauia*.[71] The eight are set in calcium. They make up two rows—four in one row, four in the other—but the rows are not alike, they bend. Here are the names of the bones in the first or upper row:

Boat bone, *iwi waapa*[72] [naviculare]
Moon bone, *iwi mahina*[73] [lunare]
Wedge bone, *iwi makia*[74] [cuneiforme]
Pea or round bone, *iwi poepoe*[75] [orbiculare]

20   The naviculare and the lunare are the ones joined with the radius and it is here that the hand turns as upon hinges. The orbiculare is on the side of the hollow of the hand and on the ulna side. Feel with your hand and you will know that it is just the radius and is plain to see at the corners of the hand.

Here is the second of the rows relating to the bones of the palm of the hand:

Quadrangle bone, *iwi ahalike*[76] [trapezium]
Irregular bone, *iwi ewaewa*[77] [trapezoid]

Large bone, *iwi nui*[78] [magnum]

Hook bone, *iwi lou*[79] [unciform]

The magnum bone has a large head and is joined with the naviculare bone and the lunare bone of the first row. The hook of the unciforme bone is for the muscles fixed there.

If someone wants to have an accurate knowledge of these bones, he must learn the true bones, *iwi maoli*,[80] bones that are joined as well as these bones that are separated.

FAN-SHAPED BONES, OR METACARPUS

These are five bones. The joint is a hinge with the wrist, and the joint with the finger bones floats. These bones and the wrist bones are wrapped very securely by ligaments, and these do not lose strength when performing duties.

HAND BRANCH BONES, OR PHALANGES

There are three bones each in the real fingers, but only two in the thumb, *manamana nui*.[81] The thumb is short and strong and it can work against the four other fingers when they all work together.

BONES OF THE LOWER LIMBS

2 twist strings on thigh bones, *iwi hilo* [femur]

2 board-in-front-of-a-canoe bones, *iwi kuapoi*[82] [patella]

2 stand-up bones, *iwi ku*[83] [tibia]

2 joined bones, *iwi pili*[84] [fibula]

14 foot protuberance bones, *iwi puupuuwawae*[85] [tarsus]

10 fan-shaped foot bones, *iwi peahi wawae*[86] [metatarsus]

28 foot branch bones, *iwi manamanawawae*[87] [phalanges]

60

21   # TWIST STRING ON THE THIGH BONE, OR FEMUR

This bone is the longest and largest of all the bones in the body. It has a large head called the hen's egg. It has a neck that is uneven, tilted, as if turning to one side. This head goes into the large cavity of the hip bone, where it rotates. Because it may get loose, it is bound by a cord. This bone has a large protuberance at the base of the neck, hence it is called the shoulder [greater trochanter]. Just below it is a very small protuberance called the small shoulder [lesser trochanter]. Its companion is the large shoulder [greater trochanter]. There is a ridge on the inside that runs from the top downward. It is rough and so is called the rough ridge. The extremity at the lower end of this bone is large and where it joins with the tibia it is spread out. This joint is a hinge.

BOARD-IN-FRONT-OF-A-CANOE BONE, OR PATELLA

This is a small, round bone secured to the muscles of the thigh at the upper border, and at the lower border there is a cord that holds fast to the tibia. When the muscles pull, the patella slips over the femur and raises the leg or foot. The patella somewhat resembles the wheel of a ship.

STAND-UP BONE, OR TIBIA

This is the third of the bones joined at the knee. Its large head is joined with the femur. It has a small protuberance to which the ligament of the patella adheres. There are two small ridges where the fibula enters, two borders, and at the end of the foot it is joined to the ankle bone [tarsus]. A protuberance at the inside of the foot secures the foot from slipping inward.

JOINED BONE, OR FIBULA

It is a long and very slender, *uuku*,[88] bone attaching on the outer side of the leg. It is joined to the tibia on the outer side a little below the knee and also at the sole of the foot. There is a protuberance at its tip outside the sole of the foot so that it prevents slipping outward. This bone is covered with pulling muscles for the sole of the foot. That is perhaps its greatest responsibility there.

22

FOOT PROTUBERANCE BONES, OR TARSUS

There are seven bones in each foot. They are:
Hinge bone, *iwi ami*[89] [heel, calcaneum, os calcis]
Block bone, *iwi kuekue*[90] [ankle bone, astragalus, talus]
Four-equal-sided bone, *iwi ahalike*[91] [cuboid]
Fish bowl bone, *iwi ipukai*[92] [naviculare]
First wedge bone, *iwi makia mua*[93] [first or medial cuneiforme]
Second wedge bone, *iwi makia lua*[94] [second or intermediate cuneiforme]
Third wedge bone, *iwi makia kolu*[95] [third or lateral cuneiforme]

If one should look at these bones, perhaps he will understand why they were put there. The calcaneum is at the opening of the bones in the foot. The astragalus lies far behind the cuboid bone and is joined together with the ankle and the third of the cuneiforme bones. The naviculare is low at the joint of the calcaneum. Its straight side is attached to the cuneiforme bones. The cuneiforme bones are set down together. Their big one is the first which adheres to the big toe bone on one side and another with the naviculare. Their small one is there in the middle called the second or intermediate cuneiforme and the third is on the outside adhering to the naviculare and the metatarsus. These bones are built up securely and are wrapped up very securely with a ligament.

FAN-SHAPED FOOT BONE
OR METATARSUS

Each foot has five fan-shaped foot bones, *iwi peahi wawae*[96] [metatarsus], each adhering to another. The big toe is not separated like the thumb of the hand. At the little toe there is a protuberance where it joins with the cuboid bone. This protuberance is for the pulling muscles.

FOOT BRANCH BONES,
OR PHALANGES

These are fourteen bones, just like the hand; however, the joints are short. There are several small bones at the pulling tendon under the big toe, four in the foot of a man, eight in another, found in some and not found in others. Thus these bones are not numbered. These bones are called seed bones, *iwi anoano*[97] [sesamoid], and their job is perhaps like that of the patella.

23   # A LIST OF NAMES OF THE BONES

1 forehead [frontal]
2 side [parietal]
1 rear [occipital]   } Bones of the head alone, 8
2 temple [temporal]
2 sieve [ethmoid]
1 bat [sphenoid]

2 upper jaw [maxilla]
2 cheek [malar]
2 nose [nasal]
2 tear [lachrymal]
2 roof-of-the-mouth [palate]   } Bones of the face, 14
2 rolled-up [turbinated]
1 partition [vomer]
1 lower jaw [mandible]

8 milk-drinking [incisors]
4 eye [canines, cuspids]
8 double [premolars, bicuspids] } Teeth, 32
8 large double [molars]
4 adult [wisdom]

1 tongue [hyoid]   Tongue, 1

2 hammer [malleus]
2 back, *hua*[98] [anvil]   } Bones of the ear, 8
2 round [orbicular]
2 stirrup [stapes]

7 neck [cervical]
12 back [dorsal]   } Vertebrae, 24
4 loin [lumbar]

1 chest [sternum]   Sternum, 1
24 side [ribs]   Ribs, 24

2 hip
1 hollow of the back [sacrum] } Pelvis is the overall name of these bones, 4
1 anus [coccyx]

2 paddle [scapula]
2 necklace [clavicle]
2 pillow [humerus]
2 cubit [ulna]
2 handle [radius]   } Bones of the upper limbs, 64
16 wrist [carpal]
10 palm [metacarpal]
28 fingers [phalanges]

24   2 thigh [femur]
2 kneepan [patella]
2 stand-up [tibia]
2 joined [fibula]   Bones of the lower limbs, 60
14 ankle [tarsal]
10 instep [metatarsal]
28 foot branches [phalanges]   Total 240

REGARDING LIGAMENTS

This is the name of the wrappings, *wahi*,[99] and the cords, *kaula*,[100] which firmly secure bones to one another as well as the protuberances and joints. They are white, bright, slippery things, and they hold fast and do not suddenly tear apart when there is pulling. There are so many ligaments that they perhaps have not all been counted. Some are different from others. However, they have a single, important purpose and that is to hold the bones firmly so as not to break loose. Some ligaments are long like ropes, others spread out, and still others resemble netting, *aa laulau*.[101]

A ligament joins the extremity at the head of a bone and another extremity at its cavity where it rotates.

Another adheres outside the protuberance, one in front, another in back, where they fit properly.

Some are placed to cross, *kau kea*,[102] each other, such as inside the knee, because these bones merely adhere. There is no shallow cavity for one bone to go inside another. Look at the ligaments that crisscross in the chicken egg [head of the thigh bone]. Cut open the patella and separate it, then the brightness and the firmness will be seen.

There is another ligament among the attached bones of the hands and the feet. This is a thin ligament, like paper. An edge is secured at the long ridge of a bone and another edge is at the ridge of its companion.

Another is a vein like ligament. All the joined bones are surrounded by these ligaments, looking like a bag, *eke*.[103] Perhaps there is fluid inside the aforementioned vein like ligament and a hard lump of fat, which lubricates, so that the moving back and forth and the shaking of the protuberances can slip and slide easily.

So, for example, when a man is working with his jacknife, *pahi pelu*,[104] and he wants the closing to be smooth, he would pour oil in it. This is the same thing. If the joint is dry, then perhaps it may be rigid.

There are other ligaments inside the body which secure the intestines and the brain. The explanation of all these things cannot be done properly.[105] Here is the thing that is clear: the skill of our Creator, because bones hold fast which are like a house made of wood in which our souls reside. Then he bound it securely with ropes.

Ligaments feel no pain should they be cut open with a knife, but should a bone joint be sprained, then the ligaments will feel pain due to their being pulled. The pain is not great in the beginning; however, if it is prolonged, then pain will increase.

REGARDING MUSCLES

[The muscles are described in nine tables in the Appendix beginning on page 65 of the translation. These tables correspond to pages 28–43 in the original Hawaiian text.]

There are many muscles inside our bodies. When counted there are 527. They are the same in all the bodies of all persons. Only a few are not the same. Take a small piece of red flesh of a cow or a pig or a chicken. Boil it in water until it is thoroughly cooked. Then open it and you will see that what belonged to the muscle is only a little and the small parts lie down together very much like the [fibers in the] native *olona*. Go further by opening the fibers, which are very fine and appear like fine hairs. Hence the fibers are called, in other words, bundles of fine hairs. A single fiber has numerous fine hairs and there are many fibers in a single muscle. The muscles are wrapped in a thin envelope. A muscle is not joined with another muscle so that when they work there is no entangling, likewise the small parts. They each have separate wrappings.

The small parts are collected at the ends [of the muscle belly] and are joined together with several cords called tendons. The tendon is like a muscle but cord like. The tendons are very firm. They will not quickly break when pulled hard. If a tendon is exposed, the fine hairs like those of the muscles can be seen, hard and firm. The hairs also lie straight; they are not twisted, are not turned over and over, and will hold fast.

26   The muscle and its tendon are the things that pull, but it is the bone that is the lever, to play up and down, when the limbs are at work. Here is the way it works: an end of the muscle is rooted on a bone. Its body is horizontal, lengthened out, and when it reaches the protuberance, the muscle becomes a cord and adheres securely to a bone. In pulling, the small muscle parts shorten until they can go no farther. The bone quickly moves because of the pulling of the cord. If the bone breaks, the muscles pull. This action moves the broken off pieces of bone alongside each other.

Therefore, the limb becomes short and very crooked. Should someone think of straightening [the bone], he must pull so that the length will be the same as it was before. Then the broken bones will be back in order and will stand upright with the other side. When this is done, wrap [the area] securely so that the bone will not slip down. Then blood will bring calcium and deposit it there in order to mend [the bone] securely.

Perhaps you should feel the muscle called the biceps. It is there when the arm flexes upward. That muscle is based at the scapula and its cord is attached to a protuberance at the head of the radius bone. If you lift your arm, the muscle will contract, the cord will pull, and the arm will move. The other side has an opposing muscle, which will make it straight. One muscle will work opposing another. That is the way the majority of the muscles work in order to return to the original place they were pulled from. The muscles' work is divided into two or more equal parts. If they worked at the same time, the limbs would not bend at all; they would just relax [stay in one position], just like the muscles of the neck that hold the head upright. Pulling of a muscle will bend [the head] forward or sideways, another will [cause it to] lean over, another will [cause it to] bow down. That is what allows a man to labor based on what he wants to do, but correct pulling occurs only when the fine hairs [fibers] are lying down.

The shapes of the muscles are many: long, short, spread out, square, triangular, circular, cross-shaped, and many other shapes. Some are large, others are small just as God created them to do heavy work sometimes, light work at other times. It is up to man to decide which of the many muscles he pulls. They are his obedient servants. They do not refuse work because of weariness, though the weariness may cause muscles to ache. If the man is not thinking of pain, the muscles will not think of that but will just work. These muscles are called helping muscles [voluntary muscles] because they obey [the will].

Other muscles are different. A man does not truly know what they do. He cannot strengthen them. They cannot remain alone quietly. A man sleeps, but they are always at work because their existence is independent; hence they are called independent [involuntary] muscles. Some are in the stomach, where they work on food. The heart is another. It opens and shuts continuously, day and night, so that blood can move to all the parts and when the blood returns and enters the heart until it is full, then it opens and shuts again and that blood flows out again. The entering [pumping] of blood is what it does, man cannot tell it to do so. The helping [voluntary] muscles are found in breathing. They work day and night, but a man can encourage them to hasten breathing. He can also stop breathing for perhaps a whole minute. In the same way the aforementoned breathing muscles [involuntary muscles] pay little attention to the man's thought, because if there is no thought, then they will work correctly, they are not lazy.

The independent [involuntary] muscles are skilled in what they do, from birth on, but the voluntary muscles do not truly know what to do when there is a newborn baby. They have to be taught. Thinking is the basis for learning. When a child is born, he stretches out his arms, perhaps strikes his nose, perhaps his nails scratch his face. He knows it hurts so he stops doing this and stretches out his arms to somewhere else. When he is a little bigger, his eyes see something he wants, a *lei*,[106] perhaps or whatever. His hands try to grab it. He tries many times to get this thing. It is the same when he rolls over, creeps, and moves. In all these activities he is being taught, then he knows.

The moving of the muscles does not end when the breath departs and death occurs. If the muscle is cut, some small indefinite muscles pull back. It is a remarkable thing to see an eel, *puhi*,[107] writhe in the fire while being broiled in ti leaves, because it is in its last moments of life with the pulling of its muscles.

The majority of muscles come in pairs, one is on the right side and the other on the left. If one is marked in this way* it is a single muscle, it has no helper, and if this mark is missing the reader must know that there is another on the other side of the body. The muscles have not all been written down in this book, there are still many more.

28

Here is another thing. In reading the catalogue below one must read from left to right: first, the name, then the place where it is based [arises from], *hoohumuia'i*,[108] and its function. All will be about that muscle. *[See table "Muscles of the Head" on pp. 66–67.]*

29   Your attention, students. These tables may be puzzling to all of you but soon some will understand when you look carefully at the drawings at the end of this book. If perhaps the muscles were cut away and separated from the body, then you will see with your eyes. That is the way to make it very clear.

Perhaps some of you might go to America. There you will see these things and perhaps when you are there you will learn everything to make you wise and perhaps you may become physicians.

30   There are eight ear muscles, which pull and shake the ears. The majority of men cannot do this, but the horse, donkey, and other animals are very skillful in doing this. *[See tables "Muscles of the Lower Jaw" and "Muscles of the Neck" on pp. 68–69.]*

31   There are three small muscles inside the ear that pull: one is attached at the handle of the malleus to strike another at its foot to raise it up again from when it struck, and the third is at the stapes and it pulls. They are independent [involuntary] muscles.

32   There are perhaps twenty-five muscles remaining in the neck. They do much work but because they are small and their real names are not known, they are not written down in this book. Some swallow, some have to do with sound, and others with the tongue. The tongue is a pulling muscle, rooted in the thick of a great number of muscles. Therefore,

33   the tongue is quick when speaking. *[See tables "Muscles Outside the Abdomen," "Muscles within the Abdomen," and "Muscles of the Chest" on pp. 70–72.]*

Four straight muscles are at the neck adhering to the spine so that they pull the head forward and to the side.

34   These are not all of the muscles of the back as written. *[See table "Muscles of the Back" on p. 73.]*

35   Some were left out so as not to confuse the students.

36–37   There are perhaps fifty muscles from the elbow and going down to and ending at the fingers, some work quickly, and some work carefully, moving back and forth. They have not all been written down. *[See tables "Muscles of the Upper Extremities" on pp. 74–75.]*

38   There are many more muscles in the hand, perhaps forty or more. There are short muscles, some rooted in the wrist, others in the palm of the hand, and some adhere to the finger bones, some at the long tendons of the muscles of the hand, in order to help them in their work.

39   Rapid succession work appropriate for the short muscles are engraving, penmanship, and blowing the bamboo. These are the many activities proper for these aforementioned muscles. Some pull to the side to turn the hand, others bend. However, their names have not been written down in this book. *"Muscles of the Lower Extremities" on pp. 76–77.]*

42   ## CONCERNING THE CIRCULATION OF BLOOD

People of Hawaii were frequently asked about their thoughts as to the movement of blood and the thoughts of the ancient people. Some had no thoughts on the movement of this thing. They supposed blood lay quietly in the flesh and when it was cut then it flowed. When the flow was heavy they believed that pain was also great. They did not know that there was blood in the vessels. Their belief was that there was air inside the arteries and because of the pulsating they thought that there was breath and life within. It was said that there was only water inside the heart, hence its name, water protuberance. Perhaps it should have been called blood protuberance. Had they looked carefully they would have seen blood inside that protuberance. That may not have been the thought of the unenlightened people of Britain in the ancient time. They looked carefully and saw blood in the vessels and it flowed when cut by a knife. But they did not understand circulation. They thought that blood rose up, in the night, from below, and that perhaps all the blood was up there in the head. When it became day the blood receded and went downward to the feet. Therefore, a man desired to lie down because the blood in his head was gone and by lying down the blood would turn around and rise up to the head, its former place. That was the thing that caused a man to rest, *hiemoe*,[109] and fall asleep, or so they thought.

In the ancient times some people cut open a corpse and looked into the heart, which was between the two lungs. They immediately thought that the heart was a very hot thing and that was why it was placed between bellows of cold air, which would abate that heat. They also believed that the pulsating was the jumping of liquid in the hot heart, which was shot into the arteries, that is, the jumping of blood, wind, air, and heat which were there inside. This period of foolishness has passed because some people in Britain have been enlightened.

In the year of the Lord 1620 Harvey published a book explaining his thought on the movement of blood everywhere inside the body. His explanation is as follows:

The heart is the source of blood. When one side [the right side] opens and shuts, blood runs into the lungs, where it branches out and joins together with the very fine branches [bronchi] of the throat [trachea], receiving and sending out air. There the blood is changed: what was black is changed into red and returns in small vessels joined into four veins called lung [pulmonary] veins. This new and good blood enters the left ear [auricle/atrium] of the heart, which quickly opens and shuts, then the blood enters the left belly [ventricle]. The left belly [ventricle] opens and shuts, and blood moves into the aorta and from there into arteries, where they branch out to the entire body. The branches are very fine and cannot be seen by the eye. Then the blood turns about in the veins and flows quietly until it reaches the right auricle of the heart, one from above, the other from below. This is black blood, which enters the ear [auricle], and the blood flows into the right belly [ventricle]. It opens and shuts and the blood moves again to the lungs. That is what Harvey explained; however, it was not embraced by educated people at the time. Some people rejected this with unkind thoughts of him, but since that time, some 200 years or more, this idea has become famous and Harvey is being counted among the wise men.

REGARDING THE HEART

If the student wants to learn fully about the heart, he must go and get a heart of a goat or perhaps that of a pig and examine it carefully because it is like that of a man.

Be very careful in cutting, as the vessels are short. Observe carefully and know those things on the outside, then cut. You will see a place bulging, on one side. Cut the ear [auricle] and proceed going underneath, then cut the second belly [ventricle], like the first, and carefully bail out the fluid. It is ready.

Observe these things in the heart:

Veins, descending/superior vena cava
Veins, ascending/inferior vena cava
Right ear [auricle/atrium]
Right belly [ventricle]
Lung [pulmonary] arteries
45   Left ear [auricle/atrium]
Left belly [ventricle]
Swollen artery [aorta]

Short arteries*
Left necklace bone artery [subclavian artery]
Left timbers on the sides of a ship, *oa*,[110] artery [left common carotid artery]
Heart [coronary] artery
Heart [coronary] vein

Observe the sides of the ventricles you have just cut open. The thick sides are the left ventricle, and the small thin sides belong to the right ventricle.

Thrust your hand into the right ventricle and go into the right auricle/atrium, from there, inside the large vein at the junction where the vein is descending and the vein is ascending, you will find an open space. Its sides are thin and the opening adheres a little for comfort. Don't be troubled if you do not find these vessels. It may be that they were cut by the knife and cut together with the side of the right auricle. Search for a small hole where the heart [coronary] vein enters. Thrust your hand into the side of the right ventricle; feel the hole there; it is for the pulmonary artery.

Feel inside the left auricle and you will find four holes for the veins entering from the lungs. Feel with your hand inside the left ventricle and you will find the hole for the aorta. These are the eight blood vessels of the heart.

THE CLOSINGS OF THE HEART

Look at the three closings at the base of the aorta, perhaps resembling valves, hence they are called valves. There are several valve closings at the base of the lung [pulmonary]

---

*This has been branched out into two: the right timbers on the side of a ship, *oa a akau*,[111] [carotid] artery and the right necklace bone artery [subclavian].

arteries, like that of the swollen artery [aorta]. The work of these closings is like that of an overseer of the pump.

Look again inside the right ventricle where some pulling muscles are placed with a great many fine cords, adhering to the three triangular flat ligaments [leaflets].

46 The ligaments [leaflets] come together at the base as a border between the ventricle and the auricle. If you find four ligaments you may think that some were cut into two in the cutting. Insert your finger under the cords, go past under a ligament [leaflet], then put together the sides that were cut. Lift the ligaments [leaflets]. Then you will see clearly the closing of these ligaments [leaflets]. These closings are called triangular closings [tricuspid valves]. There are two closings [bicuspid valves] in the left auricle/atrium [mitral valve]. However, its work and its name are the same as the right auricle/atrium. Muscles are the things that pull the ligaments [leaflets] so that the closing is perfect.

Observe the place cut by the knife and you will truly see the nature of the heart. It is a pulling muscle, but the thin muscles are not straight; rather, they entwine greatly. These are the things that allow the heart to open and shut vigorously.

When these things have been seen, you must consider the movement of the blood in the heart and the circulation throughout the body.

When the black blood descends from the head and arms and also in the rising from the legs and from the abdomen and the return of its blood to the heart, the blood is joined together in a single place. It enters the right auricle of the heart. When the auricle is full, it quickly opens and shuts and the blood goes into the right ventricle since it is opened. That is what the right auricle does, the filling up of the right ventricle, and because it is the first part of its work, its sides are thin, perhaps one and a half inches [millimeters].[112] The second part is the movement of the blood when it opens and shuts.

The right ventricle is filled with blood, it quickly opens and shuts, the tricuspid valves jump and join together, the hole is stopped up, blood cannot return to the auricle, the closing valves of the pulmonary artery are open. The blood goes straight there and is branched out to the lungs. The right ventricle expands; the closing valves are attached firmly so that blood cannot go back. This is what the right ventricle does, it moves the blood one to two feet; therefore its body is not as large as that of the left ventricle. The auricle and the ventricle work equally, *kike*.[113] One, part does not wait until the work of its companion is done; it does not hurry in doing things.

47   The left side of the heart does the same as the right side. Red blood travels from the lungs and enters the left auricle; it opens and shuts quickly and quickly drives the blood inside the left ventricle. When the blood enters, it makes the left ventricle work. It has an important job, which is to open and shut and to move the blood to the aorta and then to all the places. In its opening and shutting, the closing valves jump and shut the hole through which the blood entered. If there is no hole there and the left ventricle opens, the blood of the aorta cannot return because the closing valves are shut.

Here is another thing: the auricles work together with the ventricles. Feel the shooting in the wrist. That is the pulsating of the blood due to the opening and shutting of the left ventricle. When at rest that is the time when the auricles open and shut.

The aorta is a thing that opens and shuts to move the blood. So it is with all the arteries. They open and shut to help the heart.

It is believed that 33 pounds of blood are in the body of a man; 75 openings and shuttings in a single minute. One ounce of blood fills the heart in a single open and shut operation; 2 minutes and a half for the blood to circulate; 24

cycles in one hour; and 1056 cycles in a day and night. The left ventricle is very strong in opening and shutting, so say some learned people. It is the same as lifting 100,000 pounds! This is not easy to explain but it is very strong.

The heart is wrapped in a tight, very secure, covering. There is no hole for anything to enter it. It has an artery that carries its blood. This artery [coronary] exits at the base of the aorta and is branched out in the heart. This blood is returned inside the right auricle.

CONCERNING ARTERIES

There are several branches of the aorta. The first are two arteries for the heart. The second is the short artery that **48** branches out into two: the right carotid and the right subclavian. The third is the left carotid, the fourth is the left subclavian. The carotid artery is for the head. At the subclavian, the blood goes to the arms and to the small branches. There is a branch at the wrist, the muscle above is not big. What you feel there is the pulsating of the heart. You can also feel it in other places of the body. If the heart opens and shuts quickly, it may be due to high temperature. If [the pulse] is very rapid, it may be due to trembling [fibrillation]. If it is slow and weak, then it is clear that the opening and shutting of the heart is close to stopping and death is near.

The aorta travels and clings to the spine, goes down as far as the partition [diaphragm] between the intestines and the lungs, then the small arteries branch off for the liver and the arteries for the intestines. When the aorta comes to the fourth of the bones of the loins [lumbar region] at the [level of the] navel, it is divided into two [branches]: one goes to the right leg, the other to the left leg. There are so many branches of the arteries that if one thinks he will learn them all properly he must cut open a corpse and examine carefully. Feel your own body and if you find a pulse you are correct to think that here is an artery. It is the pounding in the ears and in the head. It is indeed the thing that throbs inside the stomach. This thing is evident in an empty stomach; therefore, one may be mistaken and think he is sick. Knowledge of arteries is an important thing to the physician because if he should cut a sick person he must not cut in ignorance or else a vessel may be wrongly severed. He may not be able to stop [the bleeding]. If an artery is cut in two, a skilled person will know exactly where to tie it off and stop the flow of blood.

THE VEINS

Where the small arteries end is the beginning of the veins. It is a continuous thing with them, small things mixing together and big things that do not branch. A vein is thin and the blood is dark when looking at a small muscle. Inside the veins are the closings that prevent the blood from going backward. If a vein is cut, the blood can stick together tightly. It will never swell up like an artery. The blood of a vein does not flow greatly when there is a small cut. It will close up between the place where it was cut and the heart. Then it will flow. Veins and arteries go together. Veins are outside, just under the skin. Arteries are not there because it would not be right for these things to be at a place where there is frequent cutting.

CONCERNING NERVES

The head is the source for thinking and thought. It is believed that the soul resides there. The brain is inside the head, wrapped by two bundles of blood vessels. Nine branches of the brain [cranial nerves] are shown in the word for the sphenoid bone. There is a large branch at the spine hole, of the occipital bone. There the spinal nerves move throughout the body. It is most important for the nerves to go together with the artery and the vein in protected places between the muscles. A nerve is like a white cord. There is no hole inside it. Its job is to know and to carry that information to the brain. Like a fisherman sitting quietly in a canoe who puts down a line, this is the same thing. If a fish is hooked, the fisherman knows quickly, as the information rises up to him through the line. If the line is cut, then he would not know that the fish is caught.[114] The spirit sits quietly in the brain. The nerve cords, which are numerous, go from the brain to all parts of the skin. If something touches the skin, the man knows quickly and that information goes up through the nerve to the brain. If the nerve is cut, the man will never know that something touched him. He is numb.

Perhaps everybody knows about numbness in the thigh when sitting crookedly for a long time. Numbness is due to the nerve being cramped and if it is tied by a cord there will be numbness because the information cannot rise to a cramped place. That is the meaning of brain sickness. It happens when the nerves are cramped, perhaps because of the swelling of a fontanel or because of the wrong rising [increased pressure] of blood in a fontanel, the thing that is cramped.

50 The soul is situated inside the body to act as a ruling master, from above. The brain is his ruling chief, *noho alii*,[115] and the nerves are his sending messengers; if not, then the arteries are the major pathways where the messengers can travel along. Here I am writing, putting down my left hand on the paper and an insect flies by and bites at my knee. The information rises immediately to the nerves and arrives in the head. Then I think of driving it away. That thought moves quickly in the nerves and reaches the muscles and tells them to pull. They do that immediately, bringing the hand down to the knee to brush away that aforementioned troublesome thing. All actions are like this: information comes and moves along the nerves, *aalele*,[116] but the person is not thinking about this. Much information comes to the eyes; the eyes see and the hands do the work, likewise the ears. Someone might call to you, the ears hear quickly, you immediately think of going there. The red muscle [Rectus femoris] and all the muscles quickly pull and it is then that the legs move. Likewise, touch and taste in the mouth. These are different kinds of information, but movement and clarity of understanding are in the nerves.

The thing we call the seat of thought, intestines, *naau*,[117] is situated in the head, not in the belly. The seat of thought and the soul are alike. But some may think differently, that the seat of thought is where the work begins and the soul is the thing that does the work. In that way thought comes from the soul. When the time comes, God will come and take the soul. That is when all activities will cease; the lungs will stop breathing; the receiving and sending out of blood by the heart will stop; the muscles will cease to pull; the eyes will shut tightly; the ears will not hear; the person will lie quietly as he becomes a corpse and quickly decays. The soul will go to God and will be either punished or rewarded according to his deeds.

The separation of the soul and the body is not forever. The two will be together again. The corpse will rise from the earth, from the ocean, or from where he was scattered, and the soul will enter into him. Then the thing spoken of in Matthew, chapter 25, verse 31, to the end of the chapter, will be done.[118]

51   CONCERNING THE ABDOMEN

There are two different places here: the chest and the abdomen. The lungs and heart are the things inside the chest. The liver, stomach, spleen, kidneys, and the urinary bladder are the things inside the abdomen.

The partition between the chest and the abdomen is a pulling muscle [diaphragm]. It adheres to the lower rib bones, the spine, and the sternum. This is a muscle for breathing. When it pulls, it is like a pump, pulling the lungs downward, then air enters through the nose, which fills the empty space [in the lungs]. When there is a fright the chest trembles. It is perhaps [due to] the shrinking back of this partition of the chest and abdomen.

The liver is on the right side [of the abdomen] under the ribs [and extends] as far up as the chest. It makes the bile inside the blood. When the black blood [venous] returns from the intestines it goes toward the heart; the veins enter into the liver and there they branch again. There the bile is separated from inside that aforementioned black blood [venous]. Then the veins join together as one, which rises up and enters the ascending veins. The bile is left inside its vessel [bile duct] until it is time for the person to eat. The bile flows and enters the stomach to be mixed with the food. The responsibility of the bile is not very clear. It is believed it is the thing that separates that which is good in the food and those things which are bad, the dregs, which are left behind.

The stomach is on the left side. It is the bag or bundle for food, *laulau*.[119] It is thin and there is much blood in the blood vessels that are on the outside. Its work is to soften the food.

The spleen is a very long internal organ adhering to the outside of the stomach. Its duties are not clear. Some people say it is a blood depository for the stomach because it holds a great amount of blood; however, it is not clearly known.

There are two kinds of intestines: the large and the small. They are all covered with a sheath that covers and holds fast the bowels. The start of the small intestine is there where the stomach ends. It is one foot long and so it is called the foot-long intestine [duodenum]. The point [duct] of the gall bladder enters at this intestine. From the duodenum to the large intestine, the length of the small intestine is four fathoms, *anana*,[120] long and about one inch in size when measured from one side to the other side. The small intestine coils and crooks around the navel, then enters the large intestine, called the colon. No other point [duct] of the intestines enters another like the small intestine enters the large intestine. A four-sided figure [appendix] enters above the head of the colon. Matter [food] moves along the small intestine to the colon. The colon's head is at the right buttocks. It rises from [near] the right kidney, turns underneath the liver and outside the small intestine as far as the left side just under the stomach, then returns underneath and goes crookedly as far as the sacrum. From there it goes down in the middle and goes out.

Here is the explanation of the movement of food from top downward. Food enters the mouth, is chewed by the teeth until ground smooth, and is mixed with the mouth's saliva, which makes the food slippery; then it goes down. The food goes from the top of the tongue over the hole in the throat, then the palate shuts the hole securely so that the food does not enter the throat. The chewed food goes down and enters the stomach. There it is mixed with the stomach fluid, which is a slippery, smooth fluid, and the flow, *hooheenee*,[121] is strong. It and the saliva that was swallowed earlier, along with the spreading out and extension of the stomach, quickly change the solid food into a liquid, which then enters the duodenum. Some of these liquified things are absorbed while in the stomach and the duodenum, and while in that state of being absorbed, they pass through five fathoms of intestines, the nutrients being consumed leaving behind the dregs. There are a great many sucking vessels [lymphatics] that insert their openings into all the intestines; the small ones, which are the most numerous, are like pig's bristles. They are filled with liquified food that resembles milk. The sucking vessels [lym-

phatics] are joined into one on the left side of the spine. Its size
is like a goosefeather; however, the placement is crooked. The
rich liquids rise until they reach the [level of the] throat, then
enter the vein of the left arm and move together with the
blood as far as the heart. From there it goes to all parts of the
body changing into muscle, bone, fat, and all things to
53 strengthen the body. This movement is constant; therefore, it
is not good for man to just sit and eat. It is proper to eat frequently, perhaps three times a day. However, it is not good to
burden the stomach wrongfully by making it work too hard
because of a great amount of food in it. The food inside the
stomach will then be heavy and bitter. This is the cause of
heartburn, sudden internal pain, heat in the stomach, nausea,
and vomiting. The stomach will not be able to work until that
bitterness is eliminated, rejected. Here are the other serious
sins: smoking tobacco and spitting out saliva. Saliva is something good to swallow, for it melts food. If tobacco smoke is
swallowed there will be bitterness. Smoking tobacco will
weaken the stomach so it cannot process food to benefit man.
The real duty of the body is to reduce [the weight of] the body,
and vegetables reduce [the weight of] the body. For example,
take a vegetable garden. Water makes vegetables grow big;
sunshine evaporates water. So if there is only water and no
sunshine, then the vegetables will be soaked, damaged. Likewise, work is good for man. Therefore, if one does not work,
he should not eat.

Look at the New Testament, the second letter of Paul to
the Thessalonians, chapter 3, verse 10 and read.[122]

The kidneys, *puupaa*,[123] are at the spine, enclosed in fat,
konahua,[124] one on the right, the other on the left, just above
the hip bones. Their job is to separate urine that is inside the
blood; therefore, blood travels there in the urinary [renal]
artery, a branch of the aorta. There are two long channels,
each ten inches long, into which urine flows and enters the

underside of the urinary bladder. Urine is a fluid in which there are also salt, calcium, and other things. There are eleven things in urine and many things go from within the body into the urine. Sometimes salt and calcium will be mixed and a hard lump may [form and] become large. It cannot come out and may grow into a large stone because of the constant mixing of calcium in the urine. That aforementioned stone, rolling around inside the urinary bladder, will become a very painful thing and a man can die in pain. Therefore, a knowledgeable person in this profession will cut into the urinary bladder, scissors will be directed inside, and the stone will be seized and taken out.

There is much fluid remaining inside the blood. Perspiration is an important thing. It comes from within the very fine artery branches and due to their being so small and fine, water just comes out, it does not come out as red blood. One source of illness is here because when a chilly wind blows or perhaps cold water touches that skin, all the openings of these blood vessels quickly adhere. The heart has to do its work with added strength to let the water out. If it cannot, then the body becomes hot; the stomach will feel dreadful due to the heat. Because the blood may be moving vigorously in the liver, much bile will be made. It is yellow. The remedies are perspiration, *puholoholo*,[125] and cathartic medicines, where heat bring will bring out fluids. There is salt in perspiration and also calcium. Another fluid is mucus, made by the arteries of the nose. Saliva from the mouth is produced by salivary glands, *anoano*,[126] below the tongue, at the joinings of the lower jaw as well as other places.

AN EXPLANATION OF THE FIGURES

Look at the letters and numbers in this book, then match the same letters in the figures for the explanation.

FIGURE I   [p. 155]

All the bones of man are collected and joined together until each is joined perfectly to another. Here are the bones seen in a front position. The letters of the alphabet point to the same letters in the drawing.

BONES OF THE HEAD

a, frontal

e, parietal

i, temporal

o, sphenoid

u, nose bone

h,h, malar

k, maxilla

l, mandible

m, neck bone

55

BONES OF THE BODY

a, vertebrae, 12

e, loin bones, 5

i,i, sternum

o, upper rib bones, 7

u,u,u, lower rib bones, 5

h, sacrum

k,k, hip bones

l, mons pubis

m,m, buttocks bone

BONES OF THE UPPER EXTREMITIES

a,a, clavicle

e,e, scapula

i,i, humerus

o,o, radius

u,u, ulna

h,h, carpus

k,k, phalanges

BONES OF THE LOWER EXTREMITIES

a,a, femur

e,e, head of the femur

i,i, patella

o,o, tibia

u,u, fibula

h,h, calcaneum

k,k, phalanges

FIGURE II   [p. 156]

In this drawing the man is turned so as to see the bones of the back.

BONES OF THE HEAD

a,a, parietal

e, occipital

i, temporal

o, malar

u, mandible

BONES OF THE BODY

a, neck bones
e, back bones
i, loins

o,o, hip bones
u, sacrum
h, coccyx

BONES OF THE UPPER EXTREMITIES

a,a, clavicle
e,e, scapula
i,i, humerus
o,o radius

u,u, ulna
h,h, carpus
k,k, phalanges

BONES OF THE LOWER EXTREMITIES

a,a, femur
e,e, tibia
i,i, fibula

o,o, calcaneum
u,u talus
h,h, phalanges

FIGURE III   **[p. 157]**

56

3
FRONTAL BONE
a,a, sinus
e,e, eye socket

i,i, nasal projection
o, temporal ridge
u,u, orbital plates

4
TEMPORAL BONE
a, scaly part [squamous part]
e, band projection [zygomatic process]
i, base of ear
o, styloid process
u, external ear opening

5
CROWN OF THE HEAD
a, clavicle
e,e, parietal bone
i, occipital bone
1,1, fontanel suture
2,2, sagittal suture
3,3, lambdoid suture
4,4, temporal suture
o, posterior fontanel
u, anterior fontanel

6
HYOID

7
BONES, *IO*,[127] OF THE EAR
1, malleus
2, anvil
3, stapes
4, stapes turned under
5, round bone, *iwi hoehoe*,[128]

8
SPHENOID BONE
1,1, large wings at the temple
2,2, small wings
3,3,3,3, the feet

FIGURE IV   [p. 158]

7
THE SPINE
1,2,3,4,5,6, nerves coming out
between the vertebrae
7, portion of the small intestine
8, coccyx
9,9, kidneys
10 liver
11 stomach

9
SCAPULA
a,a, place where it joins with
the clavicle
e,e, place of the first rib
i, place of the throat
o,o,o, at these places the
[ribs] attach
u, place where the cartilage
attaches to the sternum

8
NECK BONES
a, its body
e, branched middle projection
i, place of joining with another
bone, w,[129]
o,o, side projection
u, spinal nerve hole

10
PELVIS
a, its body
e, middle projection [process]
i,i, place they meet with
another bone
o,o, rib projections

57

FIGURE V   [p. 159]

11
JOINING OF THE HEAD
OF FEMUR
1, hip bone
2, cavity of the chicken bone
3, femur
4, head of femur
5, cord, ligament

12
SCAPULA
1, clavicle
2, sternum
3, scapula
4, humerus

13
ELBOW
1,1, radius
2,2, ulna
3,3, humerus

14
INSIDE CARPUS
1, ulna
2, radius

15
INSIDE CARPUS
1, naviculare
2, lunare
3, cuneiforme
4, orbiculare
5, trapezium
6, trapizoides
7, magnum
8, unciforme

16
METACARPUS
1, index finger
2, middle finger
4, small finger

FIGURE VI   **[p. 160]**

21
ANKLE
1,1,1, tibia
2,2,2, fibula
3,3,3, ligaments

22
METATARSUS, *kapuuwai*,[130]
1, calcaneum
2, astragalus
3, fish bowl bone, *ipuka*,[131]
4, cuboides
5, 3rd cuneiforme
6, 2nd cuneiforme
7, 1st cuneiforme

23
Toe bones

24
Big toe bones

58   **FIGURE VII**   **[p. 161]**

25 [2 in the illustration]
kneeling

26
A HAND HELD BY
LIGAMENTS
1, radius
2, ulna

27
A foot held by ligaments

FIGURE VIII [p. 162]

29

MUSCLES OF THE FACE
1, Occipito-frontalis
2, Corrugator supercilii
3, Orbicularis palpebarum
4, Levator labii superioris
   alaeque nasi
5, Levator anguli oris
6, Zygomaticus major
7, Levator labii superior proprius
8, Buccinator
9, Orbicularis oris
10,10, Depressor labii inferioris

30

1, Occipito-frontalis
2, Buccinator
3, Levator anguli oris
4, Zygomaticus major
5, Zygomaticus minor
6, Sterno-cleido mastoides
7, Parotid gland supplies mouth
   with saliva

FIGURE IX [p. 163]

31

1, Sterno-cleido mastoideus
2, Digastricus
3, Throat
4, Clavicle

32

1, Intercostales externi
2, Intercostales interni
3, Rectus abdominis
4, Pyramidalis
5, Transversalis abdominis
6, White mark

FIGURE X [p. 164]

33

1, Obturator internus
2, Iliacus internus
3, Psoas magnus
4, Border of hip bone

34

1, Platysma myoides
2, Pectoralis major
3, Pectoralis minor
4, Serratus major anticus
5, Obliquus descendens externus

FIGURE XI   **[p. 165]**

53,[132]
1, Deltoids
2, Supra spinatus
3, Infra spinatus
4, Latissimus dorsi
5, Teres major
59 6, Teres minor
7, Triceps extensor cubiti
8, Brachialis internus

36
1, Trapezius or cucullaris
2, Rhomboides
3,3, Latissimus dorsi
4, Serratus posticus inferior
5, Splenius
6,7, Large underpart of thigh

37
1, Pronator radii teres
2, Flexor carpi radialis
3, Palmaris longus
4, Flexor carpi ulnaris
5, Biceps flexor cubiti

FIGURE XII   **[p. 166]**

1,1,1,1,1,Trapezius or cucullaris
2, Latissimus dorsi
3, Deltoid
4, Infra spinatus
5, Triceps extensor cubiti
6, Sterno-cleido mastoideus

FIGURE XIII   **[p. 167]**

38
1, binding ligament
2, Extensor digitorum communis
3, Extensor minimi digiti

39
1, Abductor pollicis manus

40
1, Pronator radii teres
2, Pronator radii quadratus

FIGURE XIV   [p. 168]

41
1, Gluteus medius
2, Pyriformis
3, Leg nerve
4, Biceps flexor cruris
5, Semi membranosus
6, A nerve
8, An artery and a vein
   in between the two
9,9, Gastrocnemius

42
1, Sartorius
2,2, Rectus femoris or rectus cruris
3, Patella
4, Cruralis or cruraeus
5, Artery

43
Arteries of the fish and the heart
a, Heart

FIGURE XV   [p. 169]

44
Blood vessels and muscles
1, Straight muscles, cut
2, Sartorius
3, Rectus femoris or rectus cruris
4, An artery
5, A vein
6, A nerve

45
1, Veins
2, Artery
3, Gastrocnemius

46
Two sides of the heart, separated

60   ## FIGURE XVI   [p. 170]

47   48
The legs drawn to
see the muscles and cords
1, Binding ligament

49
The ear, *Kapepeiao*,[133]

FIGURE XVII   [p. 171]

50   51
The legs
1, Gastrocnemius
2, Plantaris

53
The eye
1, Visual nerve
2, Clear center
3,4,5, Places of the eye
6, Skull

52
Inner ear

FIGURE XVIII   [p. 172]

54
The heart
1, Descending vena cava
2, Ascending vena cava
3, Liver vein
4, Pulmonary artery
5, Pulmonary vein
6, Aorta
7, Short artery
8, Left carotid artery
9, Left subclavian artery
10, Left ventricle
11, Left auricle
12, Right auricle
X Heart vein

55
Branches of the carotid artery
The skull cut by a saw so as to
see the brain and the branches of
the brain artery, *a*.
1, Carotid artery
2,3, Zygomaticus muscles cut
    by a knife
4, Buccinator
5, Masseter

The arrows point out the movement
of the blood inside the blood vessels.

FIGURE XIX   [p. 173]

56
The brain and the cranial
nerves drawn and separated
1, Brain
2, Branches of the 5th nerve
3, Rib nerve
4, Lumbar nerve
5, Sacral nerve

57
The intestines
1, Stomach
2, Colon
3, Large intestine
4, Small intestine

APPENDIX
A CATALOG OF MUSCLES

MUSCLES OF THE HEAD

(pp. 28–31 of original text)

Name	Based at (Arises from)	Place Attached (Inserted into)	Function
Behind forehead	Ridge above the rear bone (Its spread-out cord rises over the head.)	Skin of eyebrows and base of nose, *ibo*	To pull the skin of the head up and back To raise the head
Forehead wrinkles, eyebrows	Above the root of the nose, *ibo*	Border of the Behind forehead, above the eyebrows	To wrinkle the eyebrows
Encircle eyelids	Surrounds the edge of the eye socket	Corner of the eye attaching to the nose (tear duct)	To wink and shut the eyelid
Roll open eyes	Base of the eyes, center of eye socket	Cartilage of the upper eyelids	To open the eyes
Straight above Straight below Straight inside Straight outside	Edge of the hole for the optic nerve in the center of the eye socket	Hard place of the eye (opposite each other)	To pull the eyes upward To pull the eyes downward To pull the eyes inward To pull the eyes outward
Bend above	Near the rolling eye muscle. Its tendon passes through the *belaki*, in the middle, *ono*, of the eye then attaches to	The back side of the eye	To turn the eyes downward and outward
Bend below	The inner side of the eye socket	The side of the eye opposite to bend above	To roll the eye downward and inward
Wrinkled	At the side of the base of the nose	The upper lip and the winglike projection of the nose	Raise the upper lips, dilate the nostrils
Raise up lips	Upper jaw bone under the eye socket	Middle of the upper lip	To raise the upper lip

(continued on next page)

MUSCLES OF THE HEAD (continued)

Name	Based at (Arises from)	Place Attached (Inserted into)	Function
Front crooked nose	Edge of the eye socket	Corner of the mouth	To pull the corners of the mouth upward
Middle crooked nose	Band of the temple bone	Corner of the mouth	To pull the corners of the mouth upward
Last crooked nose	Band of the temple bone	Corner of the mouth	Pulls outside and above the corner of the mouth
To blow	At the border of the bicuspids, upper and lower	Corner of the mouth, the duct of the large seeds [parotid gland] in the upper space inside this muscle	To silence the mouth
Grimace nose	Border of the lower jaw at the edge of the chin	Corner of the mouth	Pulls the corner of the mouth downward
Fold lower lip	Above the chin	Middle of the lower lip	To draw the lip downward
Encircle mouth	The spreading out of the small indefinite muscle pieces at the corner of the mouth, a small piece will move	Surrounds the mouth and joins with the small parts of that corner	To shut the mouth, project outward
Squeeze nose	At one wing of the nose and another wing	The two are joined together above the nose	To squeeze the nose

ibo: typo. *ibo* should be *ibu*.
belaki: Eng. bulbi or trochlea, resembling a pulley (*Dorland's*, 1400).
ono: center of the eye; perhaps for *onobi*.

MUSCLES OF THE LOWER JAW
(pp. 30–31 of original text)

Name	Based at (Arises from)	Place Attached (Inserted into)	Function
Temple of head	Lower edge of the parietal bone and the upper edge of the temporal bone. It enters under the bands.	The first branch of the lower jaw bone	Pulls the lower jaw upward, a very strong muscle for chewing
Chew	Upper jaw bone close to the cheek-bones and the bands.	Base of the first branch and the space of the lower jaw	Pulls the lower jaw upward, lifts and carries
Bat inside	Feet inside the sphenoid bone	Lower jaw, inner side of the space	To lift up the lower jaw
Bat outside	Feet outside the sphenoid bone	Outer side of the space of the lower jaw	To lift up the upper jaw
Long opening of the mouth	Base of the ear	The chin	Pulls the lower jaw downward and opens the mouth

MUSCLES OF THE NECK

(pp. 30–31 of original text)

Name	Based at (Arises from)	Place Attached (Inserted into)	Function
Contracting the skin	The loose skin, *alu*, at the chest muscle, *io kau*, and at the paddle muscle	The loose skin of the lower jaw and the cheeks	To pull the skin of the cheek downward
Look side to side	The head of the chest bone and the first half of the necklace bone	Protuberance at the base of the ear and in back	For the head to turn to look behind

alu: to relax, hang down.
io kau: chest muscle.

MUSCLES OUTSIDE THE ABDOMEN
(pp. 32–33 of original text)

Name	Based at (Arises from)	Place Attached (Inserted into)	Function
Lean, slant outside	Lower edge of the eight rib bones near the cartilages	White lines, *kaba keokeo waena*, of the abdomen from top to bottom and the border and the edges of hipbone	To compress, **boonou**, the abdomen, and if only a single muscle to pull it will turn the body
Lean, slant inside	Projections of the three lowest loin bones at the sacrum and the edge of the hipbone	The cartilages of the floating ribs, and the white line at the pubis and sternum	To compress the abdomen and to turn the body
Horizontal, level	Cartilages of the seven lower ribs at the side projections of the lower seven loin bones and the edge of the hips	White lines from top to bottom and the chest cartilages	To compress the abdomen
Upright, perpendicular	Chest cartilage	Pubic bone	To compress the abdomen and to bend the body downward
Stagger	Pubis	White lines below the umbilicus	To help the upright muscle

kaba keokeo waena: lit., white line. Dr. Judd's translation from Latin *linea alba*.
boonou: not in L. Andrews. To compress (Smith, 71).

MUSCLES WITHIN THE ABDOMEN
(pp. 32–33 of original text)

Name	Based at (Arises from)	Place Attached (Inserted into)	Function
Closed inside	Long circling hole of the hip-bone, the hole closed by it	Base of the great shoulder of the femur	To roll the leg outward
Four equal-sided lumbar	Edge of the hipbone, back side	The cartilages of the floating ribs, at the white line, at the pubis and sternum	To secure the spine and perhaps to turn to the side
Small line of lean flesh	Below the back bone, projection side	Mons pubis, above the cavity of the chicken egg bone	To bend forward
Big line of lean flesh	The loin bones and the lower back bone	Femur, a little below the small shoulder	To lift and raise the thigh
Inside the hip bone	On the inner side of the hip bone	Femur at the Psoas magnus muscle	To lift and raise the thigh

MUSCLES OF THE CHEST
(pp. 32–34 of original text)

Name	Based at (Arises from)	Place Attached (Inserted into)	Function
Large chest	Clavicle, sternum, and the upper seven rib bones	Space of the humerus	To draw the arm forward
Lei bone	Cartilage of the rib bones	Underside of the clavicle	To draw the clavicle forward
Small chest, *uukuu*	The third, fourth, fifth rib bones	Pointed projection of the scapula	To suspend the scapula
Front toothless	The eight superior ribs	Underside of the scapula	To pull the scapula forward
Exterior rib place	Lower edge of a rib bone lying across in front	Top edge of each rib bone	To pull the rib bones upward while working; they breathe vigorously when a man is breathing with difficulty
Interior rib place	Lower edge of a rib bone lying across in back	Top edge of each rib bone	
Chest	Middle of the sternum, internal part	The cartilages of five rib bones except the upper two	To pull down the cartilages of the rib bone in breathing

uukuu: typo. should be *uuku*.

MUSCLES OF THE BACK
(pp. 34–35 of original text)

Name	Based at (Arises from)	Place Attached (Inserted into)	Function
Back between the shoulders	The occipital bone and the spinous process, *oi waena*, of the neck- and backbones	Clavicle and scapula	To lift the shoulders and raise *aia* the head
Flat back	Edge of the hipbone, projections of the sacrum, loins, and perhaps the six backbones, adhere to the scapula	Humerus, space for the cord of the biceps	To roll the humerus and pull it backward
Lower toothless	The spinous processes of the lower backbones and the top three loin bones	Lower edge of the lower four rib bones near the cartilages	To pull the rib bones outward, downward and backward
Four-sided figure leaning back	The spinous processes of the lower three backbones and the four upper backbones	Scapula from top to bottom	To pull the scapula upward and backward. Cut in the center of two muscles
Fragment	The spinous processes of the four lower backbones and the four upper backbones	The upper two neck bones and the side of the occipital bone	To pull the head backward and to the side
First pile together	Sacrum, hipbone, and the spinous processes, rib processes, and the loin bones	Lower edge of the rib bones, a flat tendon	To draw the rib downward, to move the body and to straighten the neck
Second pile together	Like the above, a flat cord	The side projections of all the backbones and the single lower neckbone	To straighten the body

oi waena: *oi*, projection; *waena*, between [vertebrae] (Smith, 76).
aia: typo. should be *ala*.

MUSCLES* OF THE UPPER EXTREMITIES
(pp. 34–39 of original text)

Name	Based at (Arises from)	Place Attached (Inserted into)	Function
Above the scapula	Upper side of the scapula and its ridge	The head of the humerus	To lift the arm up
Below the scapula	Side of the scapula and its ridge	The head of the humerus	To roll the humerus outward
Small root	Side below the scapula	Humerus at the protuberance of the neck	To roll the humerus outward
Large root	Lower corner and lower side of scapula	Side of the groove of the humerus	To roll the humerus
Line	Clavicle and the ridge processes of the scapula	Middle of the humerus	To raise up the arm
Second line	Ridge process of the scapula	Middle of the humerus	To roll the humerus forward and upward
Concave	Edges of the scapula	Humerus at the head, *pua*, of the neck	To roll the humerus inward
Sweet potato	Two sources, one, at the pointed process of the scapula, the other at the cavity of the humerus	A protuberance at the head of the radius	To bend the arm upward
Pillow	Humerus adjoining the deltoid muscle	Chest of the ulna	To help the biceps
Three foundations	Neck of the scapula, neck and middle of the humerus	The elbow at the ulna	To straighten the arm
Joint	Protuberance outside the humerus	The elbow	To help straighten the arm
Long, hard move	Protuberance outside the humerus	Radius at the tip, close to the hand	To shake the hand and to turn the hand
Long raising up	Protuberance outside the humerus	Metacarpal bones of the index finger	To raise the palm
Short raising up	Protuberance outside the humerus	The metacarpal bone of the middle finger	To raise the fingers upward

(continued on next page)

Name	Based at (Arises from)	Place Attached	Function
Opening of fingers	Protuberance outside the humerus	All the metacarpal bones	To open up the fingers
Opening of small fingers	Protuberance outside the humerus	Second protuberance of the small finger	To open up the small finger
Raise the hand	Protuberance outside the humerus	Metacarpal bones of the small finger	To raise up the hand
Bend the hand outward	Protuberance outside the humerus and the elbow	Round bone at the edge of the hand	To bend the palm inward
Palm of hand	Protuberance inside the humerus	Bracelet ligament of the wrist and branching out to the palm ligament	To bend the hand
Bend palm inward	Protuberance inside the humerus	Metacarpus of the index finger	To bend the hand
Move bottle	Protuberance inside the humerus and the chest of the ulna	The ridge in the middle of the radius on the outside	To move the hand under the palm
Move the short radius	Protuberance inside the humerus and the ridge of the ulna	Upper and outer side of the radius	To move the hand outward and over the palm
Raise thumb	Middle of the ulna and radius	Hand bone of the thumb and wrist	To raise the thumb upward
First straightening of thumb	Middle of the ulna and the radius	First metacarpal of the thumb	To raise the thumb, *nui*, upward and outward
Second straightening of thumb	At the back of the ulna	Third metacarpal of thumb	To flex thumb upward
To indicate	Middle of the ulna	Back of the hand bone of the fore finger	To straighten the fore finger
Flex base of fingers	Protuberance outside the humerus, chest of the ulna and head of radius	Second bone of all fingers	To bunch up the hand
Flex tip of fingers	Under the chest of the ulna. (Its cords enter into the hole of the cords of the base of the fold.)	Tip of all the finger bones	To bunch up the hand
Long flex of thumb	Upper and front side of the radius	Finger bone tip of thumb	To bend the thumb
Shake four equal sides	Small finger side of the ulna, near wrist	Radius side of thumb	To move the hand under the palm

*In the original text, *iwi*, bones, was used. This should have been **IO**, muscles.

pua: typo, should be **pua.**

nui: this word is missing from Judd's book.

MUSCLES* OF THE LOWER EXTREMITIES

(pp. 38–43 of original text)

Name	Based at (Arises from)	Place Attached (Inserted into)	Function
Hollow of thigh	Edge of the hipbones at the pubis.	Rough edge of the femur near the shoulders	To raise the thigh upward
Long swell of sea	Edge of hipbone at pubis	Middle of the rough edge of the femur	To lift the thigh upward
Short swell of sea	Front of the hipbone at the branch of the pubis	Above the rough edge	To lift the thigh and to cling inward
Large swell of sea	Branch of the pubic bone	Rough edge from top to bottom	To cling to the thigh inward and to help in lifting
Shut outside	Outside of the long encircling hole	Femur at the great shoulder	To roll and pull the thigh forward
Large hamstring	Edge of hip and sacral bones	Place above the rough border	To pull the thigh downward and to roll outward
Middle hamstring	Edge and outer side of the hipbone	Great shoulder of the femur	To help the Gluteus maximus
Small hamgstring	Outer side of the hip	Base of the great shoulder	To help the Gluteus maximus
Uneven	Inner side of the sacral bone	Base of the great shoulder	To roll the thigh outward
Twins	Under part of the femur	Base of the aforementioned shoulder	To roll the thigh outward
Four equal sides at thigh	Under part of the femur	Ridge between the shoulders	To pull the thigh outward
Ligament	Corner above the hip bone	The ligament envelopes the thigh	To pull the ligament until firm
Sit squarely	Corner above the hip bone	Inner part of the tibia at knee	To guide the foot over the knee
Narrow	Pubic bone	Inner part of the tibia at knee	To bend the knee
Ocherous	Hip bone near chicken egg cavity	Upper edge of the patella	To straighten the knee
Front of the thigh	Root of the great shoulder and the rough edge of the femur	Upper and outer edge of the patella	To straighten the leg

(continued on next page)

Name	Based at (Arises from)	Place Attached (Inserted into)	Function
Back of thigh	Small shoulder and the rough edge	Upper and inner edge of the patella	To straighten the leg
Straight thigh	Small shoulder of the femur	Upper edge of the patella	To straighten the leg

Directly under this muscle is the Rectus femoris or Rectus cruris muscle. Three uneven thigh muscles, two inner and one outer.

Name	Based at (Arises from)	Place Attached (Inserted into)	Function
Hamstring cord	Under the femur	Head of the tibia, inner side	To flex the leg
Hamstring ligament	Under the femur	Head of the tibia in back	To flex the leg
Two heads	Humerus *uluna*	Head of the tibia on outer side	To bend the leg
Short	Protuberance outside the femur	Head of the tibia on inner side	To help in bending

Some of the muscles below the knee.

Name	Based at (Arises from)	Place Attached (Inserted into)	Function
Outside calf of leg	Protuberance under the femur	The two are jointed together by a single cord and attached to ankle	To pull the ankle upward and toes inward
Inside calf of leg	Head of the tibia and fibula		
Plantaris	Outer protuberance of the femur and attached blood vessels	The anklebone close to the above	To help the calves a little and to pull the blood vessels downward
Front fold	Head above the tibia	Directly above the anklebone	To raise the foot
Rear fold	Back of the tibia	Middle cuneiform, *iwi makia waena*, and navicular	To draw the foot inward
Long span	Head of the tibia and outer part of the fibula	Foot bone of the great toe	To bend the great toe downward
Short span	Outer part of the fibula	Foot bone of the little toe	To pull the outside of the foot downward

*In the original text, *iwi,* bones, was used. This should have been *IO,* muscles.

uluna. Wrong word. Should be *hilo.* Gardener, 213, 229.

iwi makia waena: should be *iwi makia lua.* Perhaps Dr. Judd translated this bone as middle cuneiform, whereas on p. 22 *iwi makia lua* is the middle or second cuneiform.

ANNOTATIONS

1. *olona.* A shrub, the bark of which dressed resembles bleached hemp or flax and is made into small cords. Hawaiian frame of reference: Hawaiians knew the *olona* and used it as cordage, which was greatly prized for its toughness. Dr. Judd uses this word to mean the tendon of a muscle of animals or men. In surgery, a ligament. *Anat.* 1:24.

2. *aa.* The small roots of trees or plants. Hawaiian frame of reference. Dr. Judd uses this word to mean the veins, arteries, and other vessels, from their resemblance to the fine roots of trees (*Anat.* 1).

3. *maloeloe.* Relax, as joints of animals. *Anat.* 1. However, an adjectival meaning for *maloeloe* is firm, substantial.

4. *oolea.* To make firm, as bones do the animal system. *Anat.* 1.

5. *loli.* A species of fish. *Anat.* 1. Hawaiian frame of reference: Dr. Judd uses the *loli* to explain how it is to be without bones.

6. *une.* The action or quality of a lever. *Anat.* 1.

7. *puna.* Lime. Hawaiian frame of reference: Hawaiians were familiar with lime from limestone, used like cement. In building Kawaiahao Church, coral blocks cut from the reef at low tide were piled up and burned in kilns on the church grounds. After several days, at the opening of the kilns, lime was shoveled out (Damon, 51).

8. *pilali.* Gum of the kukui tree. Hawaiian frame of reference: *pilali* was used to trap birds. *Kumumumu*, cartilage, something between bone and meat. Why does Dr. Judd not use *kumumumu*? Perhaps *pilali* was a more commonly used word to the Hawaiians.

9. *nao.* The grain or fibers of wood. *Anat.* 2. Hawaiian frame of reference: wood grain or fibers is used to explain what calcium looks like in a large bone.

10. *helelei.* To crumble, as dirt.

11. *maloo.* Dead, as a dried-up vegetable.

12. *hakahaka.* To be full of holes; to be hollow as a bone. *Anat.* 4.

13. *iwi lae*, lit., forehead bone.
14. *iwi hua*, lit., side bone. *Anat.* 6. *Hua* may be Judd's abbreviation for *huapoo*, lit., the side of the head.
15. *iwi hope*, lit., back bone, the skull bone at the back of the head. *Anat.* 7.
16. *iwi maha*, lit., temple bone. L. Andrews (p. 83) calls it the cheek bone, *Anat.* 7. But see *maha*, side of the head, temple, L. Andrews (p. 365).
17. *iwi kanana*, lit., sieve bone. Name of a bone in the front part of the head. *Anat.* 8.
18. *iwi opeapea*, lit., bat bone. Name of a bone in a person's head. *Anat.* 8. *Opeapea*, bat, so called from the shape of the wings being similar to the ancient sails (*pea*) of their canoes.
19. *olepe.* The name of a kind of fish resembling the *pipi. Anat.* 6. Hawaiian frame of reference: a *pipi* is an oyster.
20. *pahu.* Originally a hollow coconut or other tree with a shark skin drawn over one end and used for a drum, hence anything hollow giving a sound when struck is a *pahu.*
21. *kaua.* A war, a battle. Hawaiian frame of reference: the *iwi hua* [parietal bone] is most likely to break in battle.
22. *aalolo hoao*, lit., taste nerve.
23. *unahi.* Scales of a fish. Squamous or scaly. *American Heritage Dictionary.*
24. *oolea.* Hard, to make firm. Petrous, Latin *petrousus*, rocky. *American Heritage Dictionary.*
25. *kui.* Name for small pointed instruments, a nail, pin, spike. Styloid from stylus, the sharp pointed tool for marking or engraving. Latin *stilus. American Heritage Dictionary.*
26. *lepe.* Comb of a cock. *Crista galli*, cock's comb (Gray, 78).
27. *iokupu.* Flesh growth. Polypus, name of a disease in the nose. Polyp, a growth protruding from the mucous lining of the nose. Latin *polypus. American Heritage Dictionary.*
28. *lele.* To jump, to lead. Added meaning: overlap. Personal communication with Dr. Kathleen Durante.
29. *hoai manawa*, lit., fontanel suture. *Hoai* in anatomy, a suture, a joining; *manawa*, the anterior and posterior fontanel in the heads of young children; the soft place in the heads of infants. *Anat.* 9.
30. *hoai kaupaku*, lit., ridge of a house suture. Smith's term is *sagittal suture*, for resembling an arrow lying between the bow and string. Hawaiian frame of reference: Dr. Judd uses a ridge of a

house, as bows and arrows were not commonly used or seen by the Hawaiians.

31. *hoai ka la*, lit., the [letter] *L* suture. Lambdoid suture named from its resemblance to the Greek letter *L*, lambda.

32. *iwi owili*, lit., rolled up bone. Turbinated bone.

33. *iwi paku*, lit., partition bone. Smith calls this bone *vomer* from its resemblance to a plowshare. Perhaps a plowshare was not a familiar object to the Hawaiians. Dr. Judd's term describes the function of this bone.

34. *luauhane, luaohane*, lit., soul pit, the inner canthus or angle of the eye; the lachrymal duct perhaps. The exit point of a living person's spirit was the *lua 'uhane*, or "spirit hole." This was the inner corner or tear duct of the eye. Mrs. Pukui recalls the belief that when a person sleeps, the spirit comes out of the *lua 'uhane*. It goes on little adventures, and that produces dreams. Left undisturbed, the spirit returns from its adventures. As it enters the *lua 'uhane*, it awakens the sleeper (Pukui, *Nānā i ke Kumu*, 193).

35. *kuapoi*. Name of the board on the front part of a canoe. Hawaiian frame of reference: Dr. Judd's term describes the function of this bone in the nasal bones. Same name used for the patella in the knee. *Anat.* 21.

36. *luamaka*, lit., eye cavity. Term is not in Andrews, perhaps Dr. Judd's own word. However, see *makalua* (Andrews, L., 372), socket for the eyeball. *Anat.* 6.

37. *niho ai waiu*, lit., milk-eating teeth. Smith calls these teeth "cutting teeth." *Aiwaiu*, lit., milk eater, is the epithet of a sucking infant. Why does Dr. Judd use this term for the incisors, the permanent teeth?

38. *niho oo*, lit., mature teeth, wisdom teeth. Not in Andrews, perhaps Dr. Judd's own term.

39. typo: perhaps, *uuwa* to *uaua*.

40. *kupu*. To sprout, like a plant that grows out of the soil. Hawaiian frame of reference: Dr. Judd gives an example of the appearance of a new tooth resembling the sprouting of a plant.

41. typo: *hoawi*, perhaps *haawi*.

42. typo: *wawae*, perhaps *wawe*.

43. *iwi kua*, lit., back bone. *Kua*, name of the block of wood on which kapa was beaten; anvil of a blacksmith from its similarity to the kapa block.

44. *amara* or "Mare the armorer" was probably the blacksmith of some foreign trading vessel at the islands. The first ships that vis-

ited the islands were ships of war or of discovery and their black-
smiths were called armorers, hence the word (Andrews, L., 53;
Fornander, v. 2, 241; Kamakau, 159).

45. *keehi*. To step upon, to brace with the feet; stirrups of a saddle.

46. *noho lio*, lit., horse seat, a saddle. Around 1830, *vaqueros*,
cowhands of Mexican, Indian, and Spanish descent, came who
spoke Spanish or *español*, which led to the Hawaiian word for
cowboys, *paniolo*. They were brought to the island of Hawaii to
train Hawaiians in the handling of horses and cattle. They
brought their cowboy skills and working gear such as the spurs,
kepa, and saddle, *noho lio* (Strazer, 20, 22).

47. *aole loa e hiki ke hoakaka lea aku ma ka olelo Hawaii*, lit., (I) cannot
fully explain this clearly in the Hawaiian language. Dr. Judd
admits it was difficult for him to explain clearly the mechanism
of hearing in the Hawaiian language.

48. *iwi ka*, lit., bone near the seat. *Ka* is not listed in Andrews; however, *iwi puhaka*, the bones of the loins, is an entry in Andrews.
Perhaps Dr. Judd abbreviated *puhaka* to *ka*.

49. *puuao*. Term not found in Andrews; however, *puao*, orifice of the
womb, is in L. Andrews (p. 486). Perhaps a typo, should be *puao*.

50. *ka pou hale ma ke oa*, lit., house post goes into the rafter. Hawaiian frame of reference: a house post/rafter is used to explain the
atlas bone.

51. *ipu*. Gourd. Hawaiian frame of reference: Dr. Judd compares the
shape of the pelvis to that of the gourd.

52. *iwi papakole*. Hip bone. *Papakole*, hip, the os innominatum, the
joining of the hip bone with the socket bone.

53. *iwi kikala*, lit., the hollow of the back between the hips bone; the
name of the bone called coccyx; the hip; the buttocks; the pos-
teriors.

54. *iwi okole*, lit., anus bone or coccyx.

55. typo: *puanauweia*, perhaps *puunauweia*.

56. *iwi puukole*, lit., mons pubis.

57. *iwi lemu*, lit., buttocks bone.

58. *hua moa*, lit., chicken egg. Name of the round bone that enters
the socket of the hip. *Anat.* 16. Hawaiian frame of reference: the
head of the bone looks like a chicken's egg.

59. *iwi hilo*, lit., to twist string on the thigh bone, femur. *Anat.* 16.
When a Hawaiian is making sennit for cordage, fibers such as
those covering the nut of the coconut were spun, twisted, *hilo*, on
the thigh and plaited (Handy & Handy, 171).

60. typo: *kapai* should be *kapaia*.

61. *iwi hoehoe*, lit., paddle bone. Scapula. *Hoehoe*, paddle. Hawaiian frame of reference: the shoulder bone resembles a canoe paddle.

62. *iwi lei*, lit., necklace or lei bone. Clavicle. Hawaiian frame of reference: a lei rests upon the necklace bone [clavicle].

63. *iwi uluna*, lit., pillow bone. Humerus. Hawaiian frame of reference: the humerus is perhaps the place where one rests his head.

64. *iwi kubita*, lit., cubit bone. Ulna. *Kubita*, English for cubit, an ancient unit of measure where one cubit equaled the distance from the elbow to the wrist, sometimes to the tip of the middle finger. *Hailima*, break in the arm or the elbow, also means a cubit of measure from elbow to the tip of the fingers. Why does Dr. Judd not name this bone *iwi hailima*, which was in the *Vocabulary of Words in the Hawaiian Language* by L. Andrews, 1836?

65. *iwi kano*, lit., handle bone. Radius. Hawaiian frame of reference: *kano*, handle of an *oo*, a digging stick, also, to grasp in one's arms the forearms of another as in wrestling. Perhaps Dr. Judd used Smith's description, calling the radius handle of the hand bone. Smith 30.

66. *iwi pulima*, lit., hand protuberance bone. The wrist, or carpus.

67. *iwi peahi lima*, lit., palm bone. Metacarpus.

68. *iwi manamanalima*, lit., hand branch bone. The finger, or phalange.

69. *uala*, lit., sweet potato. Biceps. Hawaiian frame of reference: perhaps this muscle resembled the sweet potato. The biceps or large muscles of the upper arm. *Anat.* 18.

70. *iwi palaoa*, lit., whale bone. Hawaiian frame of reference: *lei niho palaoa*, whale tooth pendant, an ornament worn only by high chiefs.

71. *uahau, uhauia*. Same meaning, different spelling.

72. *iwi waapa*, lit., boat bone. Naviculare or scaphoid.

73. *iwi mahina*, lit., moon bone. Lunare or lunate.

74. *iwi makia*, lit., wedge bone. Cuneiform or wedge.

75. *iwi poepoe*, lit., round bone. Orbiculare or pisiform.

76. *iwi ahalike*, lit., quadrangle bone. Trapezium. Name of a square bone in the wrist.

77. *iwi ewaewa*, lit., irregular bone. Trapizoides. Irregular in structure, as an irregular bone. *Anat.* 4.

78. *iwi nui*, lit., large bone. Magnum.

79. *iwi lou*, lit., hook bone. Unciforme.

80. *iwi maoli*, lit., true bone. Dr. Judd may have used the word *true* for long bones found in the limbs where they form a system of levers which have to sustain the weight of the trunk. (See Gray, 33.)

81. *manamana nui*, lit., large branch. The thumb.

82. *iwi kuapoi*. lit., board in front of the canoe bone. Kneepan or patella which serves to protect the front of the leg joint (Gray, 191). *Anat.* 21.

83. *iwi ku*, lit., stand up bone. Tibia. One of the bones of the lower leg. *Anat.* 21.

84. *iwi pili.*, lit., united or joined bone. Fibula. The fibula is a slender bone placed on the outer side of the tibia with which it is connected above and below (Gray, 196).

85. *iwi puupuuwawae*, lit., foot protuberance bone. The ankle bone.

86. *iwi peahi wawae*, lit., fan-shaped foot bone. Metatarsus.

87. *iwi manamanwawae*, lit., foot branch bone. The toe, phalange.

88. *uuku*, small, little. The word *slender* is in Smith (p. 35) so Dr. Judd may have added the meaning "slender" to *uuku*.

89. *iwi ami*, lit., hinge bone. The heel or calcaneum.

90. *iwi kuekue*, lit., block bone. The talus or astragalus, Greek name for a block used in a game of chance (Smith, 36).

91. *iwi ahalike*, lit., quadrangle bone. The cuboid bone in the foot. Same name for the trapezium in the wrist.

92. *iwi ipukai*, lit., sea calabash bone. Perhaps the word should be *ipukaia*, lit., calabash for containing fish or fish bowl. The naviculare. *Iwi waapa* is also the naviculare in the wrist. Why does Dr. Judd give two different names for the same Latin name?

93. *iwi makia mua*, lit., first wedge bone. Medial or internal cuneiform.

94. *iwi makia lua*, lit., second wedge bone. Intermediate or middle cuneiform.

95. *iwi makia kolu*, lit., third wedge bone. Lateral or external cuneiform.

96. *iwi peahi wawae*, lit., fan-shaped bones of the foot. Between the instep and toes is the metatarsus, in which are five bones placed like the sticks in a fan (Smith, 36).

97. *iwi anoano*. lit., seed bone. Sesamoid bone (Smith, 37).

98. typo: *hua* should be *kua*.

99. *wahi*. That which surrounds, envelopes anything. Bands (Smith, 44).

100. *kaula*. A strong cord or tendon in the animal system. *Anat.* 25. Straps (Smith, 44).

101. *aa laulau*, lit., veinlike netting in which food was carried.
102. *kau kea*, lit., to place in the form of a cross. Cross each other (Smith, 45).
103. *eke*, bag. Hawaiian frame of reference: veinlike ligaments look like the bag part of a net.
104. *pahi pelu*, lit., jacknife. Hawaiian frame of reference: a jacknife is used to explain lubrication.
105. *aole e hiki pono ke hoakaka*, lit., can't explain clearly. Perhaps Dr. Judd could not explain clearly in Hawaiian the mechanism of ligaments so he went to his Calvinist teachings by using the metaphor of bones in the human body as building blocks of a house wherein the soul resides..
106. *lei*. A neck ornament. Hawaiian frame of reference: a *lei* is used as an example.
107. *puhi*. Eel. Hawaiian frame of reference: a *puhi* being cooked is used to explain the pulling of muscles.
108. typo: *hoohumuia'i*, perhaps *hookumuia'i*.
109. typo: *hiemoe* perhaps should be *hiamoe*, but *hiemoe* may be correct due to fast speech when *a* is pronounced *e*.
110. *oa*. Timbers in the side of a ship. Hawaiian frame of reference: Dr. Judd uses timber to describe the carotid artery.
111. typo: *oa a akau* should be *oa akau*.
112. Not inches but millimeters. Perhaps Dr. Judd thought the Hawaiians would not understand millimeter, which is 0.039 of an inch.
113. typo: *kike* should be *like*.
114. Hawaiian frame of reference: Dr. Judd uses the example of a fisherman in a canoe when a fish is hooked, that it is the nerve which carried that information to the brain.
115. *Noho alii*, lit., ruling chief. Hawaiian frame of reference: Dr. Judd explaines how messages are sent out from the brain, which is the *noho alii*, ruling chief.
116. *aalele*, wrong word, should be *aalolo*.
117. *Naau*, intestines. Hawaiian frame of reference: Hawaiians believed that the seat of thought was in the *naau*, intestines.
118. "When the son of man shall come in his glory, and all the holy angels with him, then shall he sit upon his throne of his glory."
119. *Laulau*. Hawaiian frame of reference: Dr. Judd likens the stomach to a *laulau*, lit., bundle or bag of food.

120. *anana.* A common but indefinite measure formerly used; the length of the arms and body when both arms were extended, to the ends of the longest finger; a fathom (Andrews, L., 56).

121. typo: *hooheenee* should be either *hooheehee* or *hooneenee.*

122. "For even when we were with you, this we commanded you, that if any would not work neither should he eat."

123. typo: *PUUPAA* should not be in capital letters.

124. *konahua.* The inside fat of animals. *Anat.* 53.

125. *puholoholo.* Perspiration produced by steaming leaves covering over a fire; the patient sits covered with a kapa over it.

126. *anoano.* Seeds. Perhaps Dr. Judd added salivary glands. Smith (p. 220).

127. Wrong word: *IO*, should be *IWI.*

128. typo: *iwi hoehoe* should be *iwi poepoe.*

129. typo: the letter *w* should be the word, *iwi.*

130. typo: *kapuuwai* should be *kapuwai.*

131. typo: *ipuka* should be *ipukai.*

132. typo: 53 should be 35.

133. typo: *Ka pepeiao* should be *ka pepeiao.*

Anatomia
Hawaiian Text

ANATOMIA.

HE PALAPALA IA E HOIKE AI

I KE ANO

O KO KE KANAKA KINO.

———————

Ua kakauia ma ka olelo Hawaii, i mea e ao ai na haumana o ke Kula Nui, ma Lahainaluna.

———————

OAHU:
MEA PAIPALAPALA A NA MISIONARI.
———
1838.

[3]

ANATOMIA.

O ke ano o keia olelo, *Anatomia,* oia ka olelo hoakaka i ke kino, i kona ano, a me na mea a pau i hoonohoia maloko; o na *iwi,* o na *io,* o na *olona,* o na *ami,* o na *aa,* o na *puupuu,* o na *naau,* a me na *wai.* O ia mau mea a pau, a me ka lakou hana maloko o ke kino e pono ai ke kanaka, oia ka keia palapala e hoakaka aku ai.

Aia ma na aina naauao, ua nui ka poe i ao ikaika ma ka *Anatomia,* mai ka wa kahiko mai. Ua nana pono lakou i na iwi, ua kaha i na kupapau he nui wale, a noonoo pono ka naau i ke ano o kela mea keia mea a ka maka i ike ai. Ua maopopo ka nui i keia manawa. Nolaila, mahalo ka poe naauao i ke akamai o ke Akua ka mea nana i hana, a i malama hoi i na mea kupaianaha o ko lakou kino. Aole loa e hiki ia lakou ke olelo me ka poe aia, "aohe Akua" no ka mea, ua ike pono lakou ia ia maloko o kana mau hana io. Eia hoi kekahi mea pono o ko lakou imi ana; ua loaa ia lakou ke ano o na *mai,* a me na *eha;* a ua ike i ka lapaau ana: ua akamai loa na kahuna lapaau i neia wa, aole e like mamua. O Iesu, a me ka poe hana mana no ke kokuaia mai e ke Akua, o lakou wale no ka poe i oi aku ko lakou akamai i ka lapaau ana.

NO NA IWI.

He nui ke kuleana o na iwi maloko o ke kino. Oia ka mea e *maloeloe* ai, a e *oolea* ai. Ina ua hanaia ke kanaka me ka iwi ole, e like me ka loli, pehea la e hiki ia ia ke ku ae iluna? Pehea la e hele? Pehea la e hana? He *pale* kekahi iwi; me na iwi poo e pale ai i ka lolo, a me na iwi aoao e pale ai i ke ake mama. He *une* ka nui o na iwi: e like me ka laau e mahiki ai i ka mea kaumaha, pela na iwi; a o na io ka mea e huki ai.

4   *Anatomia.*

I ka wa opiopio ua palupalu na iwi, a he olu, aole e hiki wawe ka *hai;* a i oo ke kanaka ua oolea, a i ka wa elemakule e hai pinepine no ka maloo a me ka haihai wale. O ka *puna* ka mea e oolea ai na iwi; aia i kuniia ka iwi i ke ahi, alaila e ikea ai ka puna, he keokeo, aole nae e like loa me ka puna maoli, no ka huipuia o kekahi mau mea maloko. O ka *pilali* kekahi mea maloko o na iwi. Oia kekahi kumu nui o na iwi. Eia ka mea e akaka ai ka pilali. E lawe i ka iwi uha moa, a e hookomo iloko o kekahi *acida* i huipuia me ka wai, po akolu paha ka waiho ana iloko, alaila pau ka puna i ka aiia e ka *acida*, pau ka oolea, he palupalu wale no, a he akaka, kokoke like me ke aniani kona akaka ana.

I ka hookauhua ana o ke keiki, he pilali wale no na iwi, a mahope iho lawe mai la ke koko i ka puna a waiho mawaena o ka pilali, a liuliu, ua hoomahuahuaia mai ia mea, lilo iho la ka mea palupalu i oolea, no ke komo ana o ka puna maloko. E nana aku oe i ka iwi loihi a ike i ka puka kahi e komo ai ke koko.

Ua hoomakaia keia hana, mawaena konu o ka iwi, a ina he iwi nui, aia kekahi hoomaka ana ma na aoao, hele ka puna mawaena o ka pilali e like ma ka nao o ka laau, a hookui kekahi me kekahi. Ina he iwi loihi, e waihoia ka puna mawaena a ma na poo kekahi, aole e huiia keia a oo ke kanaka, nolaila helelei na iwi loihi o ke kanaka hou ke maloo.

Ina i hai ka iwi a hoopili hou ia na wahi i hai, alaila, lawe mai ke koko i ka puna a waiho, a puni ia wahi: oia ka mea e kapili hou ai ka iwi a paa.

Ua palahalaha kekahi mau iwi, he poepoe loihi kekahi, a he ewaewa kekahi. Ua pau lakou i ka uhiia e kekahi mea lahilahi uuwa, oia ka *wahi* o ka iwi, o kona mea e nalo ai i ke kalakala, a e pahee ai i ka oni ana mawaena o na io.

Ua hakahaka na iwi loihi nui, i paa lakou aole e hai wawe, a i mama lakou, a i wahi hoi e waiho ai ka momona. Eia paha ke kuleana o ka momona maloko o na iwi. I ka

wa e mai ai ke kanaka, aole e hiki ia ia ke ai i ka ai, aole
e pono ka opu ke hoonohonoho i ka ai a lilo ia i mea e
maona ai, aka, ua lilo ia i mea awaawa a me ka wela, a
me ke nahu, maloko o kona opu: — ia manawa kiiia ae la
ua momona la, a ma ke koko e lawe aku la, a hiki i na wahi a pau o ke kino, oia ka mea e ikaika ai ke kanaka i ka
wa mai, aka i liuliu ka mai ana, pau ia momona, alaila kiiia ka momona o ke kino a puni, hiki wawe iho la ka wiwi
i ua mai la. A pau ka mai, komo hou ka ai maloko o ka
opu, lilo ia i mea e ikaika ai, alaila e hoi hou ua momona
la i laweia'ku ai mamua, a piha hou na iwi i ka momona.
No ia mau mea, e pono ke waiho i ka ai i ka manawa mai:
he hoopailua ka opu i ka ai, no ka mea ua ike ia he mea
kaumaha ka ai. Mai makau ka mai i ka pololi; ina e
hoole ka opu i ka ai, aole e make koke ke kanaka i ka pololi. Nani ka lokomaikai o ke Akua i kona hoomakaukau
ana i ka momona maloko o na iwi, i mea e ola ai ke kino
i ka manawa mai.

Alua haneri me ke kanaha iwi iloko o ke kino o kakou,
a i ke ao ana ua puunaueia i ekolu papa. 1 O na iwi o
ke poo. 2 O na iwi o ke kino ponoi. 3 O na iwi o na lala.

O NA IWI O KE POO.

He kanaonokumamakolu iwi o ke poo;

  8 iwi o ke poo ponoi a puni ka lolo,
14 iwi o ka maka,
32 niho, (ko ke kanaka makua,)
  8 iwi pepeiao,
  1 iwi alelo,
  ——
63

  Aole e like loa na poo o kanaka ke nana aku. Ua hana ke Akua, he ano okoa iki ko kekahi, a he okoa iki ko
kekahi. Pela no na maka: aole loa e loaaia na kanaka
elua, ua like loa ko laua helehelena, ke imi nui ma na aina a pau. O kekahi mau mahoe, ua kokoke like ka hio-

na, aka, ina e nana pono aku alaila ikea mai ko laua mea e okoa ai.

He mea nui i na aina naaupo ke hoololi aku i ke ano maoli o na poo o ka lakou mau kamalii i ano hou. Opa kekahi ma na aoao o ke poo e lapa ai ma na aoao: ma ka lae kekahi poe, a o ko Hawaii nei, manao la lakou o ke poo lapalapa ma ka lae a ma ka *hope*, oia ke poo maikai. Ma na aina naauao, e waiho wale lakou i na poo o ka lakou mau kamalii, me ka maikai a ke Akua i hana'i ia lakou.

NA IWI O KE POO PONOI.

1 Iwi Lae, ma ka *lae.*
2 Iwi Hua, ma na *hua* o ke poo.
1 Iwi Hope, aia o *hope* o ke poo.
2 Iwi Maha, ma na *maha.*
1 Iwi Kanana, mawaena o ka lolo a me ke kumu o ka ihu.
1 Iwi Opeapea, aia maloko, malalo o ka lolo.

IWI LAE.

Hookahi keia iwi i ka wa e oo ai ke kanaka, aka i ka hanau ana o ke keiki ua mokuia mawaena, mai luna a hala i lalo i elua iwi. He iwi lahilahi; me he olepe la kona helehelena. Aia kekahi hakahaka ma ke kihi e pili ana me na iwi ihu, mawaena o na aoao elua o ka iwi lae, o ka aoao maloko a me ka aoao mawaho. He mea keia e kani ai ka leo. No ka hakahaka ke kani ana me he pahu la. A i loaa ka mai i kapaia he ihu paa, paa iho la ka puka e komo ai ka makani iloko o ua hakahaka nei, nolaila ua kanunu ka leo. Ma keia iwi kekahi hapa o ka makalua, a ma ka aoao, he lapa no ka pili ana o ka *io maha* ka mea e huki ai ka iwi a iluna. Ma keia iwi hoi na lihi, kahi e pili ai na *kuemaka.*

IWI HUA.

He mau iwi palahalaha keia, aole nae i palahalaha maoli, he opuupuu mawaho, a he upoho maloko. O na hua o

Anatomia.   **7**

ke poo aia mawaena konu o keia iwi. He ano huinaha paha ka helehelena o ka iwi hua. Oia ka iwi nui o ke poo, a naha pinepine ia i ke kaua.

IWI HOPE.

He manoanoa keia iwi no ka pili ana o na io nui e huki ai ke poo iluna. He wahi loihi kona malalo, kahi e huiia'i me ka iwi opeapea. He puka kekahi ma ka aoao malalo, he puka nui, hookahi paha iniha ka loa o ke kahawaena o ua puka poepoe la; malaila e iho ai ka lolo ma ke kuamoo, a manamana aku la ma ke kino a pau. Ma ka lihi o ka puka nui, kekahi mau puka uuku eha, a me ka hookuina o ke poo me ka iwi mua o ke kuamoo. Ma ka puka kokoke i ka hookuina iwi, e puka aku ai ke aalolo o ke elelo. Oia ke *aalolo hoao.*

IWI MAHA.

Ua puni keia iwi i ka iwi lae, a me ka iwi hua, a me ka iwi hope, a me ka iwi opeapea. He wahi iwi ewaewa keia. O ka aoao lahilahi, ua kapaia ka *hapa umahi,* a o ka aoao manoanoa ua kapaia ka *hapa oolea:* malaila na mea lohe o ka pepeiao. He wahi oi kona e huiia me ke *apo* o ka iwi papalina mamua o ka pepeiao, a he wahi puupuu kekahi mahope o ka pepeiao, ua kapaia *kumupepeiao.* He wahi oi loihi ko keia iwi ma ka aoao malalo, hookahi paha iniha a me ka hapa kona loihi me he kui la ke ano, nolaila i kapaia kona inoa, o ke *kui.* He nui na io no ka moni ana, ka i pili ma ke kui o ka iwi maha.

He nui na puka o keia iwi. O ka *puka pepeiao mawaho.* He puka nui ia ua puni i ka lihi iwi, malaila ka pepeiao. O ka *puka pepeiao maloko.* He puka nui loa aku ia ma ka aoao hope o ka hapa oolea. Ma keia puka e komo ai ke *aalolo lohe* o ka pepeiao. He wahi puka iki ma ke kumupepeiao no kekahi aalolo e hele ana i ka papalina. Aia kekahi puka ewaewa kahi e komo ai ka lohe mai ka waha mai, i ka pepeiao. He lua kekahi ma keia iwi, kahi e hookuiia'i ka iwi a lalo. Eia kekahi, e nana i ka aoao

8   *Anatomia.*

maloko, a ike i na waha ewaewa e pili ai ka lolo, a me ke
awawa o ke aalele o ka wahi o ka lolo.

IWI KANANA.

Ua kapaia keia inoa no ka nui o na puka makalii i houia
ma keia iwi, e like me ka mea lulu pepa paha a me ke
kanana. Aia kona wahi mawaena o ke poo, malalo iho o
ka lolo, ma ke kumu o ka ihu, a mawaena hoi o na maka.
Ina paha i wawahiia na iwi o ke poo a kaawale, alaila ikea
mai ka iwi kanana. He wahi aalolo ua hoomanamanaia
a kinikini na manamana e like me ka lopi keokeo, he pokole nae, komo lakou ma na puka o keia iwi, malaila e
hele ai i ka ihu. Ua kapaia kona inoa o ke *aalolo honi,*
oia ka mea e ike ai i na mea ala ke honi aku.

He hakahaka keia, he mama, he pukapuka, i mea e kani ai ka leo, a e maopopo ai ka honi ana. He lepe kona
e ku ana mawaena o ka lolo, e like me ka lepe o ka
moa, malaila e paa ai ka paku o ka lolo. Elua wahi lau-
mania o keia iwi, no ka makalua ia mau wahi; a he paku
mawaena e ku pono ana ma ka pou o ka ihu. Elua iwi
owili, e pili ana pakahi ma ka aoao o keia paku, malaila
ke kumu o ka mai, i kapaia, o ka *iokupu.*

IWI OPEAPEA.

He pani hakahaka keia iwi no ka puniu, a ina ua hoo-
kaawaleia mawaho, ua aneane like kona helehelena me
ka opeapea, nolaila kona inoa. Ua pili keia iwi me na
iwi e ae he umikumamaha. O na wahi i kapaia na *eheu,*
aia ma ka maha, o na eheu iki aia maloko iki ae, a o
na *wawae* aia ma ka wuha, ma ka pau ana o na niho oluna: eha wawae, elua maloko, a elua mawaho. O
ka *aoao makalua,* aia ia maloko o ka makalua aoao mawaho. Aia mawaena konu o keia iwi, he mau oioi eha,
aneane like me na laau ku o ka hikiee, ua kapaia na
laau kihi, a mawaena o lakou he wahi poupou, o ka *noho
lio* kona inoa.

Aia kekahi mau puka poepoe elua malalo o na laau ki-

hi o mua, ua kapaia ka *pukanana*, no ka mea, malaila e
puka ai ke *aalolo nana* a hele i ka maka.   Mahope iki mai
na puka nui i kapaia *puka palahalaha*, eha na aalolo e puka ai ma keia puka a hele i na io kaamaka.   Mahope mai
he mau puka poepoe, a nolaila kona inoa *puka poepoe;*
malaila e puka ai ke aalolo o ka iwi a luna.   Mahope mai
olaila he pukapoepoe, he loihi nae, nolaila i kapaia kona
inoa *pukapoepoeloihi.*   Malaila hoi e puka ai ke aalolo o
ka iwi a lalo.

NO KA HUI ANA O NA IWI POO.

I ka wa e hanauia'i ke keiki he uuku na iwipoo a pau,
aole i pili pono kekahi me kekahi.   Ua waihoia ke poo
pela i hiki ai ia ke puka mai, mai kahi pilikia mai.   He
palupalu ke poo ia manawa, a i pilikia loa ka puka a ikaika loa ke nahu ana, alaila lele kekahi iwi maluna o kekahi, a hooloihiia ke poo, ua loloa a ua ololi.   Nolaila e ikea
mai ka lokomaikai o ke Akua, no ka mea ina i huipuia na
iwi ia manawa a paakiki ke poo, ina aole loa e hiki ka
hanau ana; make pu ke keiki a me kona makuwahi-
ne.   Aole i lawa na kihi o na iwipoo o ke keiki, a ua
kapaia ke kaawale, he *manawa.*   A nui ae ke keiki ulu
na iwi a pau a hui pono kekahi me kekahi, i mea e pale ai
ka lolo, a eha ole, aole nae e nalowale loa kahi e hui ai;
komo kekahi iwi iloko o kekahi, e like me na iwi olepe;
aka, hiki no ke hemo ae a kaawale.   Ua kapaia ka hui
ana o na iwi he *hoai.*   Ina ua waiho loa ia ke poo, e like
kona palupalu me ka wa i hanauia'i, ina ua pono ole ia:
hina paha ke kanaka, a kuiia mai paha ke poo, eha loa ka
lolo a make koke oia.   Mai poina kakou i ke aloha aku i
ka mea nana i hana i keia me ka lokomaikai.

No keia mau mea, ua maopopo ka lapuwale o kekahi
poe, no ko lakou makemake e hoomahuahua i ka *manawa.*
Ui lakou i ka waiu maluna, a kau no hoi ka laau i mea e
naha ai ka manawa.   Aole nae e hiki ka lakou hana ke
wawahi, aole loa ia ke ano o ka waiu e naha'i ke poo.

Eia hoi kekahi mea lapuwale.   O ka waiho wale ana o

ka manawa, aole holoiia i ka wai a pau ka lepo a me ka pe-
lapela, he kapili welu wale iho no a waiho pela.   Mai makau
i ka holoi, mai makau i ka pa aku ka lima ma ka manawa,
ina paha he hewa ia, no ke aha la e makemake oukou e
wawahi i akea ai? He palupalu no ke poo o ke keiki, aole
e pono ke pa ikaika aku ka lima maluna, aole e pono ke
hahau a me ke kui aku, aka, he mea eha ole ka welu holoi,
a me ka wai mahana, a me ke kopa, ke hana oukou i na la
a pau.

NA HUINA O KE POO.

Eha *hoai* o ke poo, elua *manawa*.

1 *Hoai manawa.*   Mai kekahi maha pii iluna o ke poo
i ka manawa, a iho ilalo i kekahi maha.   Oia ka mea e hui
ai ka iwi lae a me na iwi hua.

2 *Hoai Kaupaku.*   Maluna loa ia o ke poo, mai ka *manawa mua* i ka *manawa hope*.   Aia ma ka hui ana o na iwi
hua elua, me he kaupaku hale paha.

3 *Hoai Kala.*   Aia mahope, ma ka hui ana o ka iwi
hope me na iwi hua, mai ke kumu pepeiao pii aku la i ka
manawa hope a iho ilalo i kekahi kumu pepeiao.

4 *Hoai Maha.*   Oia ka hui ana o ka iwi maha me ka
iwi hua a me ka iwi lae.   Ua ae ka iwi maha maluna o ia
mau iwi, e like me ke pili ana o ka unahi o ka ia, pela no
kona pili ana.

1 O ka *Manawa Mua.*   Ma na kihi e hui ai na iwi
hua me ka iwi lae.

2 O ka *Manawa Hope.*   Ma na kihi e hui ai na iwi hua
me ka iwi hope.   He uuku keia, he nui ka manawa mua.

NA IWI O KA MAKA.

2 Iwi a Luna.   Ua pili pono laua i hookahi.

2 Iwi Papalina.   Ma na papalina.

2 Iwi Ihu.   Maluna o ka ihu.

2 Iwi Waimaka.   Maloko o ka makalua.

2 Iwi Kileo.   Ma ka pau ana o ke a luna maloko o ka
waha.

2 Iwi Owili.   Maloko o ka ihu.

1 Iwi Paku. Mawaena konu o ka ihu, oia ka paku.
1 Iwi a Lalo.

IWI A LUNA.

Ua hookuiia keia mau iwi i kekahi o na iwi poo, a ua
pili pu kekahi i kekahi, i ole e nauwe iki i ka ai ana i na
mea ai. O na niho o luna ua hookomoia iloko o ke kae o
keia iwi. He wahi puu hoi kona, aia maluna ae o na kihi
o ka waha, a malalo iho o ka iwi papalina: he hakahaka
koloko, a ua kapaia kona inoa ke *ana.* He wahi hakahaka keia e kani ai ka leo, e like me ko ka iwi lae. Komo
kekahi aoao o keia iwi ma ka makalua, aoao lalo a maloko, a pii kekahi oi ma ka ihu i paipai no na iwi ihu, a malaila e pili ai me ka iwi lae. He wahi puka nui ko keia
iwi, aia maloko o ka makalua, a hele i ka ihu, malaila e
kahe ai ka waimaka a komo loa i ka ihu. Elua puka makalii ma ka *luauhane,* hookahi ma ka lihi luna, hookahi ma
ka lihi lalo, oia na puka e komo ai ka waimaka, aka i ue
nui ke kanaka, aole e hiki ka wai a pau ke komo no ka
pilikia o na puka, alaila helelei mawaho ma ka papalina.

IWI PAPALINA.

Aia keia iwi mamua mai o ka pepeiao, ua hookuiia me
ka iwi maha, a me ka iwi a luna, a me ka iwi lae. O ka
hookuina me ka iwi maha, oia ke *apo* no ka *io maha,* a me
ka *io nau* e huki ai ka iwi a lalo iluna.

IWI IHU.

Hookahi iniha ka loa o keia mau iwi, ua hookuiia me
ka iwi lae, a pili pu laua, moe pono maluna o ka ihu e like
me ke kuapoi maluna o ka waa.

IWI WAIMAKA.

He mau iwi uuku loa keia. Ua like kona ano me ka
maiuu o ka manamana lima, pela ka nui a me ka lahilahi.
Aia maloko o ka luamaka, ma kekahi aoao o ka puka
waimaka. Ina ua paa ua puka la, he mea mau i ka poe
akamai ke hou i keia iwi i puka no ka waimaka.

IWI KILEO.

Alua ia mau iwi a ua pili pu laua: aia ma ka pau ana o ka iwi a luna ma ke kileo. Ua hanaia keia iwi i pale mawaena o ka waha a me ka ihu. O keia mau iwi, a me na iwi owili, a me na iwi ihu, ka i ai pinepine-ia e ka *pala.* Oia ka mai a ke Akua i haawi mai i uku hoopai no ka poe moe kolohe.

IWI OWILI.

Aia laua maloko loa o ka ihu, malaila e ulu ai ka io kupu. He mau iwi mama a he lahilahi; ua owiliia e like me ka owili pepa uuku. Ua hoomanamana hou ia na aalolo honi i puka mai ai o ka iwi kanana, a hoopalahalaia maluna o na iwi owili e like me ka punawelewele. He uuku keia iwi ma ka ihu o ke kanaka, hookahi iniha paha ka loa, aka ma ka ihu o ka ilio a me kekahi mau holoholona, ua nui loa ia. Nolaila paha ka loihi ana o ko lakou ihu, i akamai lakou i ka honi i ka lakou ai, a me ka meheu wawae o ko lakou mea e imi aku ai.

IWI PAKU.

Hookahi keia iwi, ua ku mawaena o ka ihu maloko aku o ka pou. Ua pili ia ia ka pilali paku, a ua hookuiia me me ka iwi a luna. Ku kapakahi kekahi manawa, aole iwaena konu o ka ihu.

IWI A LALO.

Ua hookuiia keia iwi me na iwi maha malalo iki ae o ke apo, aia ke ami mamua o ka pepeiao. Elua manamana o keia iwi, ma ka hookui'na kahi, a ua kapaia *mana ami.* A o kekahi aia mamua mai, ua kapaia ka *mana mua.* He puka uuku maloko o keia iwi, mai kekahi aoao o ka auwae a i kekahi, i wahi e holo ai ke aakoko a me ke aalolo a manamana aku ma na niho.

NO NA NIHO.

He kanakolukumamalua mau niho o ke kanaka, he 16

ma ka iwi a luna a he 16 ma ka iwi a lalo.   Eia ko lakou
inoa;

8 Niho ai waiu,
4 Ole,
8 Kui,
8 Kuinui,
4 Niho Oo.

Me he iwi maoli la ka niho, he oolea nae mawaho i hiki pono ke nau i na mea uuwa. I ka wa e hanauia ke
keiki, aia no na niho ma ko lakou wahi maloko o ka iwia,
o na niho mua helelei maluna, a me na niho paa malalo.
A nui ae ke keiki, eono paha malama alaila puka mai kekahi niho, me he hua kanu la ua kupu mai maloko mai o
ka lepo. Elua makahiki e kupu ai na niho helelei alaila
pau; he 20 lakou. Ma ke ono o na makahiki paha helelei kekahi niho a kupu mai ka mea hou e pani ka hakahaka. Ma ka 18 o na makahiki e kupu ai na *niho oo*, ma
ka 20 paha, nolaila i kapaia lakou na niho *oo*, a me na
niho o ka *naauao.*

Kuhi hewa kekahi poe, aia na niho i hookumuia ma ke
kumupepeiao. Aole loa pela, aole e hiki ia mea ke kolo
maloko o ka iwia a hiki i kona wahi e puka mai ai.

E hoomanao kakou i ka lokomaikai o ke Akua, i kona
haawi ana mai i ka waiu na ke keiki ma ka hanau ana: a
hiki mai ka manawa pono ia ia ke ai i ka ai, alaila hoawi
oia i na niho e nau ai i ka ai.

Eia hoi kekahi manao, he lapuwale ka manao o ka poe
aua i ka waiu, a hanai i ke keiki i kekahi mea e ae. Aole
e pono ke ukuhi i ka ai, a me ka ia, i kona manawa niho
ole. He mea make ia; aole nae e hiki wawae ka make,
aka, no ka hiki ole o ka opu ke hoonoho ia mau mea a
pau, nolaila ka hokii, a me ka wiwi, a me ke nahu, a me
ka wela, a me ka ea paha, a me ka hi. Alia ka ai a loaa
ia ia na niho, ka mea e hiki ai, alaila makaukau ka opu, a
lilo ka ai, a me ka ia i mea e ikaika ai, a i mea e nui ai ke
keiki.

14   *Anatomia.*

Eia kekahi. Mai kui wale i na niho a hemo. E waiho malie pela ma kahi i kanuia'i e ke Akua; aka, i eha, a
nauwe paha, alaila hemo.

IWI ELELO.

He wahi iwi hookahi keia, aia mawaena o na io o ke
alelo, maluna o ka puu. He like kona helehelena me ka
iwia lalo, he uuku nae, ua kokoke like me ke dala ka nui
o kona poepoe ana.

NA IWI O KA PEPEIAO.

Ewalu keia mau iwi, 4 ma kekahi pepeiao, a 4 ma ke-
kahi, he mau iwi uuku loa lakou.
Iwi Hamare, ua manaoia he like me ka *hamare.*
Iwi Kua, ua like me ke *kua* a ka Amara.
Iwi Poepoe, he iwi uuku loa, nui ka hua *makeke.*
Iwi Keehi, he like loa me ke *keehi noho lio uuku.*

I ka haalulu ana o na mea kani ma ka paku maloko o ka
pepeiao, e hukiia ke au loihi o ka hamare, a kunou iho
kona poo ma kahi poupou o ke kua, ku iho la ka welau o
ke kua ma ka poepoe, a hukiia ke kepa, a haalulu nui iho
la ma kahi i hoopalahaia'i ke aalolo lohe.   He mea kupaianaha ka lono o kakou, he pohihihi, aole loa e hiki ke hoakaka lea aku ma ka olelo Hawaii.   Ina e makemake oukou e nana i na iwi pepeiao, e huli i ke poo o ka ilio paha,
o ka bipi paha, a imi maloko loa o ka pepeiao.   He iwi
maloo ka pono, aka, ina ua kiola pinepine ia ma o a ma o,
e pau paha na iwi i ka helelei; a i loaa, ua like me ko ke
kanaka.

NA IWI O KE KINO.

He kanalima kumamakolu iwi i kapaia no ke kino;
            24 Iwi Kuamoo,
            24 Iwi Aoao,
             1 Iwi Umauma,
             4 Iwi Ka.
            ———
            53

Anatomia.   15

O keia mau iwi 53, oia ke kumu e pili ai na lala, a me
ka mea e malu ai na mea palupalu, hiki wawe ka eha ke
pale ole ia i ka mea oolea.   Maloko o ke kuamoo ka hooloihi ana o ka lolo, i kapaia ke *aalolo kuamoo.*   Maloko o
ka umauma ke *ake* a me ka *puuwai.*   Maloko o ka iwi ka
ke *koana mimi,* a me ka *puuao.*

NA IWI KUAMOO.

He 24 lakou: 7 o ka *ai,* 12 o ke *kua,* a 5 o ka *puhaka.*
A ua hookuiia lakou kekahi i kekahi a paa loa.   Ina e
lawe oe i ka iwi kuamoo a nana pono aku, e ike oe i na *oi*
ekolu, elua ma na *aoao,* hookahi *mawaena konu,* eha wahi
e pili pu ai me kekahi iwi, elua maluna elua malalo, a me
ke *kino* o ka iwi, he wahi poepoe ia.   E nana i ka puka
nui no ke aalolo kuamoo, e iho ana a e manamana ana mawaena o na iwi elua a pau; pela wale no mai luna a lalo.
O na wahi oi, no ka pili ana o na io a me na olona, e huki
ai i ke kino a ku pono iluna, a e hoea hou ke kulou iho
ilalo.   He mea pilali uwauwa mawaena o na iwi e pili pu
ana, oia ka mea e hiki ai ke kuamoo ke pelu iki ai aole e
hai.
Ina e anaia ke kiekie o ke kanaka i ke kakahiaka, a
hana ikaika oia ia la a po, a ana hou ia; alaila e akaka ai
kona emi ana hookahi iniha paha ka emi ana.   Eia ka
mea e pokole ai, o ke ku ana iluna a me ka huki ikaika
ana o na io, oia ka mea e kaomi iho ai maluna o ka mea
uwauwa, lahilahi iki iho la ia, a pokole iho la ke kuamoo.
Ua hookuiia ka iwi mua o ka ai me ke poo; he ami ia
no ka hookunou ana.   Ua auwahaia, a komo mai ma ka
auwaha kahi oi o ka lua o na iwi, e like me ke komo ana
o ka pou hale ma ke oa.   Mawaena o laua ka hooluliluli
ana o ke poo, a me ka alawa ana ae.

IWI AOAO.

He 24 keia mau iwi, he 12 ma kekahi aoao, a he 12 ma
kekahi, ua like hoi ko ke kane a me ko ka wahine.   Ua hookuiia kekahi poo ma ka iwi *kua* o ke kuamoo a pela na iwi

16   *Anatomia.*

kua he 12, Ua hookuiia kekahi poo ma ka iwi *umauma,* he
pilali ko ia poo i mea e olu ai, e hiki pono ai ke hanu.   O
na iwi 7 oluna ka i pili pono me ka iwi umauma, a o na
iwi elua i koe ua pokole mai a lewa wale maloko o ka io.

Ina e hanu mai ke kanaka, piha mai la ke ake mama,
a pii mai la na iwi aoao, a hanu aku, hoi hou na iwi aoao
ilalo, a pela e upa mau ai ke kea paa i ka po a me ke ao
a pau ke ola ana.

IWI UMAUMA.

He wahi iwi mama keia; hookahi iniha a me ka hapaha
kona laula, a he umi iniha kona loa i kekahi manawa.
Ma kahi i huiia'i me na iwi *lei* kona wahi palahalaha.   He
pilali ka aoao malalo ma ka houpo.   Ua 5 paha iwi o ka
umauma i ka wa kamalii, a oo ke kanaka e hui lakou i 3
paha, a ma kekahi manawa he hookahi wale no.

NO NA IWI KA.

Oia ka inoa nui o na iwi okoa eha i huipuia, a no ka
poepoe ana ua hoohalikeia me ka ipu.   He mau iwi paa
keia, o ke kumu hoi e noho ai ke kino, a me ke poo, a me
ka lala maluna.

        2 Iwi Papakole,
        1 Iwi Kikala,
        1 Iwi Okole.

IWI PAPAKOLE.

Alua iwi ewaewa keia; ua huipuia laua ma ke alo; a ma
ke kua ua huipu me ka iwi kikala, aka ma ka olelo ana
ua puunauweia laua i pakolu na iwi.   O ka iwi palahalaha ma ka papakole ua kapaia, iwi papakole.   O kahi e
hui ai laua ma ke alo, iwi *puukole,* a o kahi e noho iho ai ke
kanaka ma ka noho,—iwi *lemu* kona inoa.   Ua kaawale
keia mau iwi i ka wa kamalii a oo ke kanaka e huiia
lakou ekolu i hookahi.   Aia ko lakou wahi e hui ai
ma ka lua o ka *huamoa* no ka iwi *hilo,* elua hapalima o ia

lua no ka iwi papakole, elua hapalima no ka iwi lemu, a
hookahi hapalima no ka iwi puukole. He kae kalakala maluna o ka iwi papakole kahi e pili nui ai na io, ua kapaia
ka *lihi*. Ma ka pau ana o ka lihi ma ke alo, elua wahi
puu, ua kapai ka mea oluna, kihi oluna, a o ka mea malalo iho, kihi olalo o ka iwi papakole. Aia mawaena o
ka iwi lemu a me ka iwi puukole he puka nui, ua kapaia,
puka poailoihi, a o kahi e hui ai ia mau iwi ua kapaia kauwahi, ka *lala* o ka iwi puukole, a o ke kauwahi, ka lala o
ka iwi lemu. He palahalaha ka papakole o ka wahine, a
he palahalaha ole ko ke kane.

IWI KIKALA.

He aneane huinakolu elua aoao like kona ano, ua huliia ka huina oi malalo. He iwi hookahi keia, aka, i ka wa
kamalii ua elima paha. Ua nui na puka maloko ona, he
umi paha, kahi e puka mai ai na manamana o ke aalolo
kuomoo.

IWI OKOLE.

Ua pili keia ma kahi oi o ka iwi kikala a ua hoo-
keekeeia maloko. He hookahi keia iwi i ke kanaka, he
elua paha, aka, ua kinikini ma na holoholona, a ua kapaia
he huelo.

NA IWI O NA LALA.

He kanaonokumamaha iwi o na lala oluna, a he kana-
ono o na lala olalo. He palua wale no lakou, ua like ko
kekaki aoao me ko kekahi aoao.

NA IWI O KA LALA OLUNA.

2 Iwi Hoehoe,	} Iwi Poohiwi.
2 Iwi Lei,	
2 Iwi Uluna,	
2 Iwi Kubita,	} Iwi loihi.
2 Iwi Kano,	
16 Iwi Pulima,	
10 Iwi Peahi lima,	} Iwi uuku a me ka poepoe.
28 Iwi Manamanalima.	

64

2*

18   *Anatomia.*

IWI HOEHOE.

He wahi iwi palahalaha keia, a he lahilahi, me he huinakolu la ke ano, e lewalewa ana mawaena o na io o ke poohiwi, aole i pili me kekahi iwi, o ka iwilei wale no. Elua
wahi oi o keia iwi. O ka *oi lapa* oia kahi e huiia me ka
iwi lei, a he *lapa* kona malaila aku a hele loa i kela aoao
o ka iwi. O ka *oi nuku*, aia ma ka aoao oloko, he palena
ia no ka iwi uluna o poholo ae maloko; o ka oi lapa ka
palena maluna, mawena o ua mau oi la he wahi lua uuku
no ke poo o ka iwi uluna, kahi e kaa ai ia iwi.

IWI LEI.

Ua hoomoeia mawaena o ka iwi umauma a me ka iwi
hoehoe ma ka poohiwi, oia kekahi mea e paa ai ka hookuina poohiwi. O ka pono nui o ka iwilei he koo, e koo ai
ka poohiwi i ole e haule mamua a malalo, a ina ua hai keia
iwi alaila haule koke ka poohiwi ilalo. He aalele nui
malalo o ka iwi lei.

IWI ULUNA.

He loihi keia iwi, a he pololei, he poo poepoe kona maluna, kahi i hookuiia'i me ka iwi hoehoe, a ua palahalaha
iki ae ma ka welau malalo, kahi e komo ae iloko o ka iwi
kubita. Me he ami maoli la keia puupuu, aole loa e kaa e
like me ka poohiwi: pelu mai no iluna a hoopololeiia hoi
ilalo, oia ka pau loa o kona wahi e oni ai.

O na hookuina iwi e hiki pono ke kaa, he poo ko lakou
a me ka lua e kaa ai, ua kapaia ia mau hookuina, he *hookuina* lewa, aka, i hiki ole ke kaa—he pelu aku a he pelu
mai, oia wale no kona—ua kapaia he *hookuina ami.* He
hookuina lewa ko ka iwi uluna ma ke poohiwi, a he hookuina ami, ma ke kuekue lima.

He wahi awawa ko luna o keia iwi no ke kaula o kekahi io, *uala* ka inoa, oia kekahi mea e pelu mai ai
ka lima, a he puu ma kela aoao keia aoao o ua
awawa la, kahi e paa ai na io e kaa ai ka lima. He lapa
loihi kekahi mawaena, no na io no. Ma ka palahalaha
malalo, he *puu mawaho*, a he *puu maloko.* E nana pono i

Anatomia.   19

ka hookuiana me ka iwi *kubita* i kahi lua e komo ai ke
kuekue, a he lua uuku iho ma ke alo no ka pepeiao mua o
ka iwi kubita.   E nana hoi i kahi e huipu ai me ka iwi
kano.   Alua iwi *loihi* i koe no ka lima.   Ua hoomoe like
ia laua, ua pili ma na poo, a ua like ko laua nui.

IWI KUBITA.

O kubita ka inoa o keia iwi, no ka mea, oia ke ana i ka
wa i ana ai ka poe kahiko i ke kubita.   Mai ke kuekue a
i ka puu e pili ai keia iwi me ka pulima, hookahi ia kubita.   Ua hooloihi kekahi poe i ke kubita a i ka welau o
ka manamana loihi o ka lima.   O ka welau o keia
iwi e pili ana me ka iwi uluna, ua like me ka iwi palaoa
paha kona helehelena, o ka elelo oia ke *kuekue*, a o ka
umauma, oia kahi e paa ai ka iwi o poholo mamua, a ua
kapaia ka *pepeiao mua* o ka iwi kubita.   O ke poo uuku o
keia iwi ua pili i ka iwi kano, a pili uuku paha me na iwi
pulima.

IWI KANO.

Ua pili ke poo uuku o ka iwi kano me ka aoao o ka iwi
kubita, ma ke kuekue lima, e like me ke pili ana o ke kubita ma ke kano, ma ka pulima.   I ka olapa ana o ka lima,
kaa aku kekahi poo, a kaa mai kekahi poo, a kaa kea ia na
iwi, aia ka lima ma ka iwi kano a huli pu me ia i ka olapa
ana.   O ka hoohiki ana ma na walu, aole ia he pono, no
ka mea, he 12 iwi malaila.

NO KA PULIMA.

Ewalu mau iwi ewaewa iloko o ka pulima, ua hahau pu
ia me ka pilali, e like ka uahau ana paha me na pohaku
ewaewa i uhauia i ka puna a paa.   Elua papa o lakou, 4
ma kekahi papa, 4 ma kekahi, aole nae i like na papa, he
keekee.   Aia ka papa mua e pili ana maluna, eia ko
lakou mau inoa;

Iwi Waapa,
Iwi Mahina,
Iwi Makia,
Iwi Poepoe.

O ka iwi waapa, a me ka iwi mahina ka i hookuiia me ka iwi kano, malaila hoi e ami nui ai ka lima. Aia ka iwi poepoe ma ka aoao poho lima a me ka aoao kubita. E haha aku oe a ike, he iwi pili wale no ia, a he akaka ma ke kihi o ka lima.

Eia ka lua o na papa e pili ana i na iwi o ka *peahi lima.*

Iwi Aha like,
Iwi Ewaewa,
Iwi Nui,
Iwi Lou.

He poo nui ko ka iwi nui a ua hookuiia me ka iwi waapa a me ka iwi mahina o ka papa mua. O ka lou o ka iwi lou, no na io ia mea, malaila e paa ai.

Ina e makemake kekahi e ike pono i keia mau iwi e pono ke ao ma na iwi maoli i hookuiia, a me na iwi kaawale.

IWI PEAHI LIMA.

Elima keia poe iwi. He ami ka hookui ana me ka pulima, a he lewa ka hookui ana me na iwi manamana-lima. O keia mau iwi, a me na iwi pulima, ua wahiia e na olona paa loa, oia ka mea e hemo ole ai ke ikaika ka lawelawe ana.

IWI MANAMANA LIMA.

Pakolu keia mau iwi i na manamanalima maoli, aka, elua wale no ko ka manamana nui. He pokole ka manamana nui, a ikaika no hoi i hiki ia ia ke ku e i na manamana eha, i ka manawa e hana pu ai lakou.

NA IWI O KA LALA OLALO.

2 Iwi Hilo,
2 Iwi Kuapoi,
2 Iwi Ku,
2 Iwi Pili,
14 Iwi Puupuuwawae,
10 Iwi Peahiwawae,
28 Iwi Manamanawawae.
———
60

Anatomia.   21

IWI HILO.

Ua oi aku ka loa a me ka nui o keia iwi i ko na iwi a pau o ke kino. He poo nui kona, o *huamoa* kona inoa, a a he ai hoi ua kapakahi me he aluli la. Komo keia poo iloko o ka lua nui o ka iwi papakole, malaila e kaa ai: a no ka hemo paha ua hikiia i ke kaula. He puu nui ko keia iwi ma ke kumu o ka ai, nolaila ua kapaia he *poohiwi*, a malalo iki ae he puu uuku iki iho, ua kapaia *poohiwi iki*, a o kona hoa *poohiwinui*. He lapa kekahi ma ka aoao maloko, mai luna a hala i lalo, a no ke kalakala ua kapaia, *lapa kalakala*. He nui ka welau malalo o keia iwi, a he palahalaha no ka hookui ana o ka iwi ku. He ami keia hookui ana.

IWI KUAPOI.

He iwi poepoe uuku keia, ua paa i na io o ka uha ma ke kae maluna, a ma ke kae malalo, he olona ka mea e paa ai i ka iwi ku. A huki na io, pahee ka iwi kuapoi maluna o ka iwi hilo, a hoala aku la ka wawae. Ua aneane like ka iwi kuapoi me ke pokakaa o ka moku.

IWI KU.

O ke kolu keia o na iwi i huiia ma ke kuli, ua hookuiia kona poo nui me ka iwi hilo. He wahi puu uuku kona, kahi e pili ai ke olona o ka iwi kuapoi; he wahi lua iki ma ka aoao kahi e komo ai ka iwi pili: elua lapa; a ma ka welau kapuwai ua hookuiia me na iwi puupuu wawae. Aia kona puu ma ka aoao maloko o ke kapuwai, oia ka mea e paa ai ka wawae i poholo ole ai maloko.

IWI PILI.

He iwi loihi a he uuku hoi, e pili ana ma ka aoao mawaho o ka wawae, ua pili i ka iwi ku ma ka aoao mawaho, malalo iki o ke kuli, a ma ke kapuwai hoi kekahi; o kona welau ka puu mawaho o ke kapuwai, i mea e poholo ole ai mawaho. Ua paapu keia iwi i na io huki no ke kapuwai oia paha ka nui o kona kule ana malaila.

IWI PUUPUUWAWAE.

Ehiku o keia mau iwi ma ke kapuwai hookahi.

Iwi Ami,
Iwi Kuekue,
Iwi Aha like,
Iwi Ipukai,
Iwi Makia mua,
Iwi Makia lua,
Iwi Makia kolu.

Ina e nana aku kekahi i keia mau iwi, alaila maopopo paha ko lakou wahi e waiho ai. O ka iwi *ami*, aia ma ka auwaha o na iwi wawae, o ka iwi *kuekue*, aia loa mahope o ka iwi *ahalike* ua pili pu me ke kuekue, a me ke kolu o na iwi makia, o ka iwi *ipukai*, aia kona poupou ma ka iwi ami, a o kona aoao pololei e pili ai me na iwi makia. E waiho pu ana na iwi *makia*, o ko lakou mea nui oia ka *mua* e pili ana me ka iwi manamana nui kekahi aoao, a o kekahi me ka iwi *ipukai*, o ko lakou mea iki aia mawaena, oia ka *lua*, a o ke kolu aia mawaho mai, a pili hoi me ka iwi *ipukai* a me na iwi *peahi*. Ua uhauia a paa keia mau iwi a ua wahiia i ke olona a paa loa.

IWI PEAHI WAWAE.

Elima iwi peahi no ke kapuwai, ua pili kekahi me kekahi, aole kaawale ka manamana nui e like me ko ka lima, a o ka manamana iki ua puu ma kahi e pili ai me ka iwi ahalike, no na io huki keia puu.

IWI MANAMANA WAWAE.

He umikumamaha iwi, e like me ko ka lima, he pokole nae na pona.

Aia kekahi mau iwi uuku ma ke kaula huki ilalo o ka manamana wawae nui, eha ma ka wawae o kekahi kanaka ewalu ma kekahi, aia i ka loaa ana, a ma kekahi aole e loaaia, nolaila aole i heluia keia mau iwi. *Iwi anoano* ka inoa o keia mau iwi, a ua like paha ka lakou oihana me ka ka iwi kuapoi.

Anatomia. 23

HE PAPA INOA O NA IWI.

1 Iwi Lae,	
2 Iwi Hua,	
1 Iwi Hope,	
2 Iwi Maha,	Na iwi o ke poo ponoi he 8.
1 Iwi Kanana,	
1 Iwi Opeapea,	

2 Iwi A Luna,	
2 Iwi Papalina,	
2 Iwi Ihu,	
2 Iwi Waimaka,	
2 Iwi Kileo,	Na iwi o ka maka he 14.
2 Iwi Owili,	
1 Iwi Paku,	
1 Iwi A Lalo,	

8 Niho Ai Waiu,	
4 Ole,	
8 Kui,	Na niho he 32.
8 Kui Nui,	
4 Niho Oo,	

1 Iwi Elelo,   O ka iwi elelo he 1.

2 Hamare,	
2 Hua,	Na iwi o ka pepeiao he 8.
2 Poepoe,	
2 Keehi,	

7 Iwi Ai,	
12 Iwi Kua,	Na iwi o ke kuamoo he 24.
4 Iwi Puhaka,	

1 Iwi Umauma,   O ka iwi Umauma 1.

24 Iwi Aoao,   O na iwi aoao he 24

2 Iwi Papakole,	
1 Iwi Kikala,	Iwi Ka ka inoa nui o keia
1 Iwi Okole,	mau iwi he 4.

2 Iwi Hoehoe,	
2 Iwi Lei,	
2 Iwi Uluna,	
2 Iwi Kubita,	
2 Iwi Kano,	Na iwi o ka lala o luna he 64
16 Iwi Pulima,	
10 Iwi Peahi lima,	
28 Iwi Manamanalima,	

2 Iwi Hilo,	
2 Iwi Kuapoi,	
2 Iwi Ku,	
2 Iwi Pili,	Na iwi o ka lala o lalo he 60.
14 Iwi Puupuuwawae,	
10 Iwi Peahi wawae,	Pau loa, 240
28 Iwi Manamanawawae,	

NO NA OLONA.

Oia ka inoa o na wahi, a me na kaula e paa ai na iwi kekahi me kekahi, a me na puupuu, a me na ami. He mau mea pahee lakou, he keokeo, he hinuhinu, a he paa loa no hoi, aole e moku wawe i ka huki ana. Ua nui loa na olona aole paha i heluia. He ano okoa ko kekahi, a he ano okoa ko kekahi, hookahi hoi oihana nui o ka hana paa i na iwi i hemo ole ae. He loihi kekahi olona, me he kaula la, he palahalaha kekahi, a he aa laulau ke ano o kekahi.

O kekahi olona ua pili kekahi piko ma ke poo o kekahi iwi, a o kekahi piko ma kona lua e kaa ai.

Ua pili kekahi mawaho o ka puupuu; mamua kekahi, a mahope kekahi, aia no ma kahi e pono ai ke hoopaa.

Ua kau kea kekahi, aia maloko o ke kuli, no ka mea, he pili wale no ia mau iwi, aole lua poupou e komo ai kekahi iwi maloko o kekahi. E nana i na olona kau kea ma ka iwi moa, e oki aku i ke kuapoi a kaawale alaila ikea mai he hinuhinu a he paa.

Aia kekahi olona mawaena o na iwi pili o ka lima, a me ka wawae, he olona lahilahi keia me he pepa la. Ua paa kekahi lihi ma ka lapa loihi o kekahi iwi, a o kekahi lihi hoi ma ka lapa o kona hoa.

He olona aa kekahi. Ua hoopuniia na hookuina iw a pau i keia mau olona, e like me ka eke. He wai paha maloko o ua aa la, a me ka haku konahua. Oia ka mea e hinu ai, i pahee ke ami ana a me ka luli ana o na puupuu.

Nolaila paha ka hana ana o ke kanaka i ka pahi pelu, ke makemake oia e olu ke pelu ana, ninini iho la oia i ka

Anatomia.   25

aila maloko, pela keia. A ina paha e maloo, alaila ma-
locloe.

Aia kekahi mau olona maloko o ke kino e paa ana i na
maau, a me ka lolo, aole e hiki pono ke hoakaka ia mau
mea a pau, eia ka mea akaka, o ke akamai o ko kakou
mea nana i hana, no ka mea, paa na iwi, oia ka laau
hale e noho ai ko kakou uhane, alaila hoa i ke kaula a
paa.

Aole e eha na olona ke kaha i ka pahi, aka i okupe ka
hookuina iwi, alaila e eha na olona, no ka huki ana o lakou; aole nae e eha nui i kinohou, a liuliu paha alaila ma-
huanua ka eha.

NO NA IO.

He nui loa na io maloko o ko kakou kino: ua heluia he
elima haneri me ka iwakalua kumamahiku. Ua like hoi
lakou ma na kino a pau o kela kanaka keia kanaka, he
kakaikahi ka like ole. Ina e lawe oe i ka mamala io ulaula o ka bipi paha, o ka puaa paha, o ka moa paha, i hoo-
lapalapaia i ka wai a moa lea, alaila wehe ae, e ike aku
oe, he maawe ko ka io a ua hoomoe like ia na maawe me
he olona maoli la. E hiki pono ia oe ke wehe hou ae i na
maawe a makalii loa a ikea mai he *heu* wale no. Nolaila
ua kapaia ka maawe (ma kekahi olelo ana) he *pupu heu.*
He lehulehu loa na heu ma ka maawe hookahi, he nui
wale hoi na maawe ma ka io hookahi. Ua wahiia na io i
ke aa lahilahi i pipili ole kekahi io me kekahi io, i hihia
ole hoi ka hana; a pela no na maawe, he wahi okoa ko
lakou, pakahi ka wahi o lakou a pau.

Ua houluuluia na maawe ma na piko, a kui pu me kekahi mea olona hinuhinu, ua kapaia kona inoa he *kaula.*
He wahi hoi ko ke kaula e like me na io, he olona nae.
Ua paa loa na kaula, aole e moku wawe ke huki ikaika
ia. Ina e weheia kekahi kaula, e ikea na heu e like me
ko na io, he oolea nae a he paa; ua moe like na heu, aole
e hiloia aole e hiliia, aka he paa no.

O ka io a me kona kaula ka mea e huki ai, o ka iwi hoi ka *une* e mahiki ai ke lawelawe na lala. Eia hoi ke ano o ka hana ana; ua hookumuia kekahi welau o ka io ma kekahi iwi, moe aku la kona kino a loihi aku hiki paha ma ka puupuu, lilo iho la ka io i kaula, a pili a paa ma kekahi iwi. I ka huki ana ume iho la na maawe io a puku mai la; lele koke ka iwi no ka huki ana o ke kaula. Ina ua haloke ka iwi a hai paha, huki na io, a oia ka mea e holo ai kekahi hakina iwi ma ka aoao o kekahi, a nolaila pokole ka lala a keekee loa: a ina e manao kekahi e hoopololei, e pono ia ia ke huki a like ka loihi me ka wa mamua, alaila hooponopono i na hakina iwi a ku pono kekahi me kekahi. A pau ia, alaila wahi a paa i mea e paholo ole ai ka iwi, a na ke koko no e lawe mai i ka puna a waiho malaila i mea e kapili ai a paa.

E haha paha oe ma ka io i kapaia ka *uala*, a pelu mai ka lima iluna. Ua hookumuia kela io ma ka hoehoe, a pili kona kaula ma kahi puupuu ma ke poo o ka iwi kano. Ina e hapai oe i kou lima puku mai la ka io, huki hoi ke kaula a lele mai la ka lima. He io ku e ko kela aoao, i mea e hoopololei ai, hana ku e kekahi io i kekahi, pela wale no ka nui o na io, i mea e hoi hou ai kahi i hukiia, e like mamua: he kike ka lakou hana ana. Ina e hana pu aole e pelu iki na lala, he maloeloe pu wale iho no, e like me na io o ka ai e ku pono ai ke poo. He kiwi kekahi huki ana, he hio kekahi, a he auwi kekahi, oia ka mea e hiki ai ke kanaka ke lawelawe mamuli o kona makemake, aka he pololei wale no ka huki ana ma ka moe ana o na heu.

He nui loa na helehelena o na io, he loihi, he pokole, he palahalaha, he ahalike, he huinakolu, he poai, he pea, ia ano aku, ia ano aku; he nui kekahi, he liilii kekahi, e like a me ka hana a ke Akua i haawi mai ai na lakou, he hana nui paha, he hana uuku paha. Aia no i ka manao o ke kanaka ka huki ana o ka nui o na io. He mau kauwa hoolohe lakou nona; aole lakou e hoole i ka hana no ka maloeloe, he eha nae ke maloeloe, aka, i manao ole ke kanaka ma ka eha, aole e manao lakou ma ia mea, e hana

aku no. Ua kapaia keia poe io, *io kokua* no ka hoolohe
ana o lakou.

He ano e ko kekahi mau io, aole e ike pono ke kanaka
i ka lakou hana ana, aole hoi e hiki ia ia ke hooikaika,
aole e hiki ke waiho a noho malie. Hiamoe ke kanaka
hana mau lakou, no ka mea, he kuokoa ko lakou noho
ana; nolaila ua kapaia lakou *io kuokoa.* Aia kekahi ma ka
opu. O ka ai ka lakou mea e hana'i. O ka *puuwai*
kekahi. E mau kona upa ana i ka po a me ke ao i mea e
holo ai ke koko ma na wahi a pau, a i hoi mai ke koko a
komo iloko o ka puuwai a ua piha, alaila upa hou, a kahe
hou aku ua koko. O ke komo ana o ke koko oia ka mea
e hana'i oia, aole loa e hiki i ke kanaka ke olelo aku. O
na io kokua i ka hanu ana kekahi, ua hana lakou i ka po
a me ke ao, aka e hiki ke kanaka ke hooikaika ia lakou a
wikiwiki ka hanu, e hiki hoi ke umi a paa ka hanu a hala
paha ka *minute hookahi.* Pela e hoolohe iki ai ua mau io
hanu la i ka manao o ke kanaka, aka i manao ole malaila,
e hana pono no lakou aole e molowa.

Ua akamai na io *kuokoa* i ka lakou hana, mai ka hanau
ana mai, aka, aole e ike pono na io kokua i ka wa kino
hou, ua aoia lakou, o ka manao ke kumu e ao ai. A i hanauia ke keiki mawaho, kikoo ae oia i kona lima, a ku i
ka ihu paha, a wauwau paha na maiuu i ka maka; a ike
oia he eha, oki iho la ia hana ana a kikoo na lima ma kahi e. A nui iki ae ike ka maka i kona mea e makemake
ai, o ka lei paha, heaha la? hoao iho la ka lima i ka lalau
aku, a hoao pinepine hiki ia mea ia ia. Pela ka huli ana,
a me ke kolo, a me ka hele, a me na hana a pau, aia i aoia alaila ike.

Aole e pau koke ka oni ana o na io ke lele ka hanu a make loa. Ina i kahaia ka io, eeke mai la kekahi mau maawe
io. He mea nui ia i ka puhi ke panau mai maloko o ke
ahi i ka lauwalu ana, no ke koena ola maloko o na io huki.

He papalua ka nui o na io; ma ka aoao akau kekahi, a
ma ka aoao hema kekahi. Ina i hoailonaia kekahi penei, *

hookahi ia io, aole ona kokoolua, a i ole keia hoailona e
pono ka mea e heluhelu ana ke manao, aia kekahi ma kela aoao o ke kino.   Aole e pau na io i ke kakauia ma
keia palapala, ua nui no nae.
Eia kekahi mea.   I ka heluhelu ana o ka papa hoike
malalo iho nei, he pono ke heluhelu mai ka hema a i ka
akau; o *ka inoa* mua, alaila *kahi e hoohumuia'i*, a mahope
mai, e heluhelu i *kahi e pili ai*, a o *kana hana* ka mea e
pau ai ia io.

HE PAPA HOIKE NO NA IO.

NA IO O KE POO.

Ka inoa.	*Kahi e hookumuia'i.*
Ohopelae.*	Ma ka lapa oluna o ka iwi hope. (Pii kona kaula palahalaha iluna o ke poo.)
Pukupukukuemaka.	Maluna ae o ke kumu iho.
Poailihilihi.	A puni ke kae o ka maka-lua.
Kaakaamaka.	Kumu maka, mawaena konu o ka makalua.
Pololei maluna. Pololei malalo. Pololei maloko. Pololei mawaho.	Kae o kahi puka no ke aalolo nana mawaena o ka makalua.
Auwioluna.	Kokoke i ka io kaakaa-maka. Puka kona kaula ma ka belaki ma ka ono o ka maka, alaila pili ma
Auwi olalo.	Aoao maloko o ka maka-lua.
Mimino.	Ma ka aoao o ke kumu o ka ihu.
Hoopinana lehelehe luna.	Iwi a luna malalo o ka makalua.
Hooewanuku mua.	Kae o ka makalua.
Hooewanuku waena.	Apo o ka iwi maha.

Anatomia.   29

Auhea oukou e na haumana. E pohihihi auanei keia
papa ia oukou, aka, e maopopo no kekahi ke nana pono
oukou ma na kii ma ka pau ana o keia palapala. Ina
paha i kahaia a kaawale na io ma kekahi kino a nana maka aku oukou oia ka mea e akaka lea ai.

Aia paha e holo kekahi o oukou ma Amerika, malaila e
ike ia mea, a malaila paha e ao i kela mea a i keia mea, e
akamai ai ia a e lilo paha i kahuna lapaau.

HE PAPA HOIKE NO NA IO.

NA IO O KE POO.

Kahi e pili ai.	*Kana hana.*
Ka ili o ke kuemaka a me ke kumu ihu.	E huki ai ka ili o ke poo iluna a i hope. E hooanuu-nuu ai ke poo.
Ka lihi o ka ohopelae ma-luna o ke kuemaka.	Hoopuku i na kuemaka.
Ke kihi o ka maka e pili ana i ka ihu, (o ka lua uhane.)	E amo ai a e hoopili ai i na maka.
Pilali o ka lihilihi o luna.	E kaakaa ai ka maka.
Wahi oolea o ka maka. (ku e kekahi i kekahi.)	E huki iluna ka maka. E huki ilalo ka maka. E huki maloko ka maka. E huki mawaho ka maka.
Ka aoao hope o ka ma-ka.	E leha ai i ka maka ilalo a iwaho.
I ka aoao o ka maka e ku e ana i ka auwi o luna.	E kaa ai ka maka malalo a maloko.
Ka lehelehe luna, a me ka loha ihu.	O ka hoaaka.
Mawaena o ka lehelehe luna.	O ka hoopinana lehelehe luna.
Kihi o ka waha.	Huki iluna ke kihi o ka waha.
Kihi o ka waha.	Huki iluna ke kihi o ka waha.

30 *Anatomia.*

Ka inoa.	Kahi e hookumuia'i.
Hooewanuku hope.	Apo o ka iwi maha.
Puhi.	Ma ka palena mai o na kui nui maluna a malalo.
Haikaikanuku.	Kae o ka iwi a lalo, lihi auwae.
Pelu lehelehe lalo.	Maluna o ka auwae.
Poaiwaha*	I ka hihi ana o na maawe io ma ke kihi o ka waha holo aku kekahi maawe a
Opa ihu.	Ma kekahi loha ihu, a me kekahi loha.

Ewalu io mawaho o ka pepeiao, e huki ai a e luli ai ka pepeiao, aole nae e hiki i ka nui o kanaka ke hana ia mea, o ka lio a me ka hoki, a me kekahi mau holoholona ka i akamai loa.

NA IO O KE A LALO.

Maha.	Lihi lalo o ka iwi hua, a me ka lihi luna o ka iwi maha. Komo ae malalo o ke apo.
Nau.	Iwi a luna kokoke i ka iwi papalina, a ma ke apo.
Opeapea oloko.	Wawae oloko o ka iwi o-peapea.
Opeapea owaho.	Wawae owaho o ka iwi opeapea.
Oakaloihi.	Kumu pepeiao.

NA IO MA KA AI.

Eeke.	Ka alu ma ka io kau a me ka hoehoe.
Alawa.	Poo o ka iwi umauma a me ka hapalua mua o ka iwi lei.

Anatomia. 31

Kahi e pili ai.	*Kana hana.*
Kihi o ka waha.	Huki iwaho a iluna ke kihi o ka waha.
Kihi o ka waha. Ua komo ka auwai o na anoano nui ma ka lewa maloko o keia io.	E mumu ai ka waha.
Kihi o ka waha.	Huki ilalo ke kihi o ka waha.
Mawaena o ka lehelehe lalo.	E pelu i ka lehelehe ilalo.
Poai ka nuku a pili me na maawe o kela kihi.	E poi ai ka nuku a e hooi iwaho.
Pili pu laua maluna o ka ihu.	E opa i ka ihu.

Ekolu io liilii maloko o ka pepeiao e huki ai, aia kekahi ua pili ma ke au o ka hamaie, e kui iho ai, a o kekahi ma kona wawae e hooala hou mai, mai ke kui ana, a o ke kolu aia ma ke keehi e ume ai oia.   He mau io *kuokoa* lakou.

NA IO O KE A LALO.

Mana mua o ka iwi a lalo.	Huki iluna ke a lalo. *He io ikaika loa i ka nau ana.*
Kumu o ka mana mua, a me ka lewa o ke a lalo.	Huki iluna ka iwi a lalo, a me ka hoolewa.
Iwi a lalo, aoao maloko o ka lewa.	E hoolewa ai i ka iwi a lalo.
Aoao maloko o ka lewa o ke a lalo.	E hoolewa i ke a lalo.
Ka auwae.	E huki ai ilalo ke a lalo, a e oaka ai ka waha.

NA IO MA KA AI.

Ka alu o ke a lalo a me ka papalina.	E huki ai ilalo ka ili o ka papalina.
Puu ma ke kumu pepeiao, a mahope mai.	E alawa ai ke poo.

32   *Anatomia.*

He iwakaluakumamalima paha io i koe ma ka ai.   He
nui ka lakou hana ana, aka, no ka liilii o lakou, a no ka
maopopo ole ma ka clelo maoli, aole i kakauia lakou ma
keia palapala.   No ka moni ana kekahi o lakou, no ka leo

NA IO MAWAHO O KA OPU.

Ka inoa.	*Kahi e hookumuia'i.*
Hio mawaho.	Lihi lalo o na iwi aoao ewalu e kokoke ana i na pilali.
Hio maloko.	Na *oi waena* o na iwi puhaka lalo ekolu, ma ka iwi kikala, a me ka lihi iwi papakole.
Iliwai.	Na pilali o na iwi aoao lalo ehiku, ma na oi aoao o na iwi puhaka lalo ehiku, a me ka lihi papakole.
Kupono.	Pilali umauma.
Kuoi.	Puukole.

NA IO MALOKO O KA OPU.

Pani oloko	Puka poai loihi o ka iwi papakole, ua paniia ka puka ia ia.
Ahalike puhaka.	Lihi iwi papakole aoao hope.
Uhao uuku.	Iwi kua lalo, oi aoao.
Uhao nui.	Na iwi puhaka a me ka iwi kua o lalo.
Papakole maloko.	Aoao maloko o ka iwi papakole.

NA IO MA KE KEA PAA.

Kau nui.	Iwi lei, iwi umauma, a me na iwi aoao luna ehiku.
Iwilei.	Pilali o ka iwi aoao luna.
Kau uukuu.	Ke kolu, ka ha, a me ka lima o na iwi aoao.

Anatomia.   **33**

kekahi, no ke alelo kekahi.   He io huki ke alelo, ua hookumuia i ka hihi ana o na io he nui loa, nolaila ka mama
o ke aleio i ka olelo ana.

NA IO MAWAHO O KA OPU.

Kahi e pili ai.	*Kana hana.*
Kaha keokeo waena o ka opu, mai luna a lalo, a me ka *lihi* o ka iwi papakole.	E hoonou ai i ka opu, a ina hookahi wale no io e hu-ki ai e huli ai i ke kino.
Na pilali o na iwi aoao lewalewa, ma ke kaha wae-na, ma ka puukole a me ka iwi umauma.	E hoonou ai i ka opu, a e huli i ke kino.
Kaha keokeo waena, mai luna a lalo, a me ka pilali umauma.	E hoonou ai i ka opu.
Iwi puukole.	E hoonou ai i ka opu, a e hookulou ai i ke kino.
Kaha keokeo waena ma-lalo o ka piko.	E kokua i ka *io kupono.*

NA IO MALOKO O KA OPU.

Kumu o ka *poohiwi nui,* o ka iwi hilo.	E kaa ai ka wawae ma-waho.
Iwi puhaka, a me ka iwi aoao lewa o lalo.	E paa ai i ke kuamoo, a e huli paha i ka aoao.
Iwi puukole, maluna ae o ka luahuamoa.	E kulou ai.
Iwi hilo malalo iki ae o ka poohiwi iki.	E kaikai i ka uha.
Iwi hilo ma kahi o ka uhao nui.	E kaikai i ka uha.

NA IO MA KE KEA PAA.

Awawa o ka iwi uluna.	E huki mai ka lima ma-mua.
Aoao lalo o ka iwi lei.	E huki ai ka iwi lei ilalo.
Iwi hoehoe oi nuku.	E lewa ai ka hoehoe.

34 *Anatomia*.

Ka inoa.	*Kahi e hookumuia'i.*
Nihomole mua.	Na iwi aoao luna ewalu.
Kulana aoao mawaho.	Lihi lalo o kekahi iwi aoao, moe kea ma ke alo.
Kulana aoao maloko.	Lihi lalo o kekahi iwi aoao, moe kea ma ke kua.
Umauma.	Mawaena o ka iwi umauma, aoao maloko.

Eha io pololei ma ka ai e pili ana i ke kuamoo i mea e huki ai ke poo imua, a i ka aoao.

NA IO O KE KUA.

Hokua.	Iwi ohope, a me na oi waena o na iwi ai a me na iwi kua.
Palahalaha kua.	Lihi o ka iwi papakole, na oi o ka iwi kikala, a me na iwi puhaka a me na iwi kua aono paha, pili hoi i ka hoehoe.
Nihomole lalo.	Na oi waena o na iwi kua lalo elua, a me na iwi puhaka luna ekolu.
Huinaha hio kua.	Na oi waena o na iwi ai lalo ekolu, a me na iwi kua luna eha.
Apana.	Na oi waena o na iwi ai lalo eha, a me na iwi kua eha oluna.
Uhau mua.	Iwi ka, iwi papakole, me na oi waena a me na oi aoao o na iwi puhaka.
Uhau lua.	E like me ka mua, he kaula palahalaha.

Aole i pau loa na io o ke kua i ke kakauia.

O NA IWI O KA LALA OLUNA.

Hoehoeluna.	Aoao oluna o ka iwi hoehoe a me kona lapa.

Anatomia.   35

Kahi e pili ai.	*Kana hana.*
Iwi hoehoe aoao o lalo.	E huki ai ka hoehoe mamua.
Lihi luna o kekahi iwi aoao. Lihi luna o kekahi iwi aoao.	E huki ai na iwi aoao iluna, i ka hana ana, hanu ikaika lakou ke naenae ke kanaka.
Na pilali o na iwi aoao elima, koe elua maluna.	E huki ai na pilali iwi aoao ilalo, i ka hanu ana.

NA IO O KE KUA.

Iwi lei, a me ka iwi hoehoe.	E lewa ai ka poohiwi, a e aia i ke poo.
Iwi uluna, awawa no ke kaula o ka io uala.	E kaa ai ka iwi uluna a e huki ai i hope.
Lihi lalo o na iwi aoao lalo eha, e kokoke i na pilali.	E huki ai i na iwi aoao iwaho, a i lalo, a i hope.
Iwi hoehoe, mai luna a lalo.	E huki ai ka hoehoe iluna a i hope. Ua moku mawaena konu i elua io.
Na iwi ai luna elua, a me ka aoao o ka iwi ohope.	E huki ai ke poo i hope, a ma ka aoao.
Lihi lalo o na iwi aoao, he kaula palahalaha.	E huki ai na iwi aoao ilalo, e hoeu ai i ke kino, a e hookupono i ka ai.
Na oi aoao o na iwi kua a pau, a me ka iwi ai lalo hookahi.	E hookupono ai i ke kino.

Ua waihoia kekahi i pohihihi ole ai ka haumana.

O NA IWI O KA LALA OLUNA.

Ke poo o ka iwi uluna.	E hapai ka lima iluna.

36   *Anatomia.*

Ka inoa.	*Kahi e hookumu ia'i.*
Hoehoelalo.	Aoao o ka iwi hoehoe a me kona lapa.
Mole nuku.	Aoao lalo o ka iwi hoehoe.
Mole nui.	Kihi lalo a me ka aoao lalo o ka iwi hoehoe.
Kaha.	Iwilei, a me ka oi lapa o ka iwi hoehoe.
Kahalua.	Oi lapa o ka iwi hoehoe.
Upoho.	Na kae o ka iwi hoehoe.
Uala.	Elua kumu, aia kekahi ma ka oi nuku o ka iwi hoehoe, a o kekahi ma ka lua no ka iwi uluna.
Uluna.	Iwi uluna ma ka pili ana o ka io kaha.
Kumukolu.	Ai o ka iwi hoehoe, a me ka iwi uluna ma ka ai a mawaena.
Kuekue.	Puu mawaho o ka iwi uluna.

He kanalima paha mau io, mai ke kuekue lima a hala loa i ka pau ana o na manamana, he hana wikiwiki ka keka-

Olapa kano loihi.	Puu mawaho o ka iwi uluna.
Hoalaloihi.	Puu mawaho o ka iwi uluna.
Hoala pokole.	Puu mawaho o ka iwi uluna.
Mohala manamana lima.	Puu mawaho o ka iwi uluna.
Mohala lima iki.	Puu mawaho o ka iwi uluna.
Hooala peahi.	Puu mawaho o ka iwi uluna.
Pelu peahi owaho.	Puu maloko o ka iwi uluna, a me ke kuekue.

Anatomia.   37

Kahi e pili ai.	*Kana hana.*
Ke poo o ka iwi uluna.	E kaa ai ka iwi uluna iwaho.
Iwi uluna ma ka puupuu o ka ai.	E kaa ai i ka iwi uluna iwaho.
Aoao o ke awawa o ka iwi uluna.	E kaa ai ka iwi uluna.
Mawaena o ka iwi uluna.	E hapai ka lima iluna.
Mawaena o ka iwi uluna.	E kaa imua a iluna ka iwi uluna.
Iwi uluna, ma ka pua o ka ai.	E kaa ai ka iwi uluna maloko.
Kahi puu ma ke poo o ka iwi kano.	E pelu mai ai ka lima iluna.
Umauma o ka iwi kubita.	He kokua no ka io uala.
Ke kuekuelima ma ka iwi kubita.	E hoopololei i ka lima.
Ke kuekue lima.	E kokua i ka hoopololei i ka lima.

hi he akahana ka kekahi, he olapa mai, he olapa aku.
Aole e pau lakou i ke kakauia.

Iwi kano ma ka welau kokoke i ka lima.	E olapa aku ai i ka lima a e huli iluna ka poho lima.
Iwi manamana o ka lima kuhi.	E hoala i ka peahi lima.
Iwi peahi o ka lima loihi.	E hoala iluna.
Na iwi manamanalima a pau.	E mohala ai i na manamana lima.
Puupuu lua o ka lima iki.	E mohala ai i ka lima iki.
Iwi manamanalima o ka lima iki.	E hoala i ka peahi iluna.
Iwi poepoe ma ke kihi o ka lima.	E pelu i ka peahi iloko.

4

38   *Anatomia.*

Ka inoa.	*Kahi e hookumuia'i.*
Poholima.	Puu maloko o ka iwi uluna.
Pelu peahi oloko.	Puu maloko o ka iwi uluna.
Olapa omole.	Puu maloko o ka iwi uluna, a me ka umauma o ka iwi kubita.
Olapa iwi kano pokole.	Puu mawaho o ka iwi uluna, a me ka lapa o ka iwi kubita.
Hooala lima nui.	Mawaena o ka iwi kubita a me ka iwi kano.
Hoopololei mua o ka lima nui.	Mawaena o ka iwi kubita a me ka iwi kano.
Hoopololei lua o ka lima nui.	Iwi kubita ma ke kua.
Kuhi.	Mawaena o ka iwi kubita.
Pelu kumu manamanalima.	Puupuu o loko o ka iwi uluna, umauma o ka iwi kubita, a me ke poo o ka iwi kano.
Pelu welau manamanalima.	Malalo ae o ka umauma kubita. (Komo kona mau kaula ma ka puka o na kaula o ka pelu kumu.)
Pelu loihi o ka lima nui.	Iwi kano aoao luna ma ke alo.
Olapa ahalike.	Iwi kubita aoao manamana iki kokoke i ka pulima.

He nui na io i koe no ka lima, he kanaha paha lakou, he keu aku paha.   He mau io pakole, ua hookumuia kekahi ma ka pulima, a o kekahi ma na iwi peahi, a ua pili ma na iwi manamana kekahi, a o kekahi ma na kaula loihi o na io o ka lima, i mea e kokua ai ia lakou ma ka lakou hana.

NA IO O KA LALA OLALO.

| Hena. | Lihi o ka iwi papakole, ma ka puukole. |

Anatomia.   39

Kahi e pili ai.	*Kana hana.*
Olona kupee o ka puupuu lima, a manamana aku i olona poho lima.	E pelu ai ka lima.
Iwi manamana o ka lima kuhi.	E pelu ai i ka lima.
Ka lapa mawaena o ka iwi kano, aoao mawaho.	E olapa mai i ka lima ilalo ka poho.
Iwi kano aoao maluna a mawaho.	E olapa i ka-lima mawaho a iluna ka poho.
Iwi peahi o ka lima nui, a me ka pulima.	E hoala i ka lima nui iluna.
Iwi manamana mua o ka lima nui.	E hoala i ka lima iluna a iwaho.
Iwi manamana kolu o ka lima nui.	E pelu ai ka lima nui iluna.
Iwi peahi o ka lima kuhi.	E hoopololei i ka lima kuhi.
Ma ka iwi lua o na manamana a pau.	E puupuu ai i ka lima.
Na iwi manamanalima a pau ma ka welau.	E puupuu ai i ka lima.
Iwi manamana welau o ka lima nui.	E pelu ai ka lima nui.
Iwi kano aoao manamana nui.	E olapa mai ka lima ilalo ka poho.

O na hana wikiwiki ka i ku pono loa i na io pokole, o ke kahakaha, o ke kakau lima, a me ke puhi ana o ka ohe, oia kekahi mau hana ku pono i ua mau mea io nei. He huki aoao ko kekahi e kiwi ai ka lima, he pelu ko kekahi. Aole nae i kakauia ko lakou inoa ma keia palapala.

NA IO O KA LALA OLALO.

Lapa kalakala o ka iwi hilo, kokoke i na poohiwi.	E hapai i ka uha maluna.

Ka inoa.	*Kahi e hookumuia'i.*
Kahela loihi.	Lihi o ka iwi papakole, ma ka puukole.
Kahela pokole.	Alo o ka iwi papakole, ma ka lala o ka puukole.
Kahela nui.	Lala o ka iwi puukole.
Pani owaho.	Mawaho o ka puka poai-loihi.
Lemu nui.	Lihi o ka papakole, a me ka iwi kikala.
Lemu waena.	Lihi a me ka aoao mawaho o ka papakole.
Lemu uuku.	Aoao mawaho o ka papakole.
Kapakahi.	Aoao maloko o ka iwi kikala.
Mahoe.	Iwi lemu.
Ahalike uha.	Iwi lemu.
Olona.	Kihi oluna o ka iwi papakole.
Hoahaaha.	Kihi oluna o ka iwi papakole.
Ololi.	Iwi puukole.
Alaea.	Iwi papakole, kokoke o ka lua huamoa.
Alo uha.	Kumu o ka poohiwi nui, a me ka lapa kalakala o ka iwi hilo.
Kua uha.	Poohiwi uuku a me ka lapa kalakala.
Pololei uha.	Poohiwi uuku o ka iwi uha.

Malalo pono keia io i ka io alaea.

Kaula lemu.	Iwi lemu.
Olona lemu.	Iwi lemu.

Anatomia.   . 4.

Kahi e pili ai.	*Kana hana.*
Mawaena o ka lapa kalakala o ka iwi hilo	E hapai i ka uha maluna.
Maluna o ka lapa kalakala.	E hapai i ka uha a e hoopili mai iloko.
Lapa kalaknla mai luna a lalo.	E hoopili mai i ka uha iloko, a e kokua i ka hapai ana.
Iwi hilo ma ka poohiwi nui.	E kaa a e huki i ka uha mamua.
Kahi oluna o ka lapa kalakala.	E huki i ka uha malalo a e kaa mawaho.
Poohiwi nui o ka iwi hilo.	E kokua i ka lemu nui.
Kumu o ka poohiwi nui.	E kokua i ka lemu nui.
Kumu o ka poohiwi nui.	E kaa ai i ka uha mawaho.
Kumu o ua poohiwi la.	E kaa ai i ka uha mawaho.
He lapa mawaena o na poohiwi.	E huki ai i ka uha mawaho.
Ke olona e wahi ana i ka uha.	E huki i ke olona a maloeloe.
Aoao maloko o ka iwi ku, ma ke kuli.	E kaikai i ke kapuwai maluna o ke kuli.
Aoao maloko o ka iwi ku, ma ke kuli.	E pelu i kuli.
Iwi kuapoi lihi luna.	E hoopololei i ke kuli.
Iwi kuapoi lihi luna a mawaho.	E hoopololei i ka wawae.
Iwi kuapoi lihi luna a maloko.	E hoopololei i ka wawae.
Iwi kuapoi lihi luna.	E hoopololei i ka wawae.

Ekolu io ololo uha, elua maloko, hookahi mawaho.

Poo o ka iwi ku aoao maloko.	E pelu i ka wawae.
Poo o ka iwi ku aoao mahope.	E pelu i ka wawae.

4*

42   *Anatomia.*

Ka inoa.   Kahi e hookumuia'i.
Poolua.   Iwi uluna.

Pokole.   Puupuu mawaho o ka iwi
                           hilo.
        Kekahi o na io malalo o ke kuli.
Oloolo wawae mawaho.   Na puupuu lalo o ka ⎫
                           iwi hilo.   ⎪
                                                   ⎬
Oloolo wawae maloko.   Poo o ka iwi ku a me   ⎪
                           ka iwi pili.   ⎭
Libini.   Puupuu mawaho o ka iwi
                           hilo a me ke aa hookuina.
Pelu mua.   Poo maluna o ka iwi ku.

Pelu hope.   Iwi ku aoao mahope.

Kikoo loihi.   Poo o ka iwi ku, a me ka
                           aoao mawaho o ka iwi pili.
Kikoo pokole.   Iwi pili aoao mawaho.

NO KA POAI ANA O KE KOKO.

Ua ninau pinepine ia na kanaka o Hawaii nei, i ko lakou manao i ka holo ana o ke koko, a me ka manao o ka
poe kahiko, aole i loaa he manao ko kekahi i ka holo ana
o ia mea. Kuhi lakou he moe malie ke koko maloko o
ka io, a i mokuia alaila kahe; a i nui ke kahe ana, manao
iho la lakou ua nui hoi ka eha. Aole lakou i ike he koko
maloko o na aa, o ko lakou manao he makani ko loko o
aalele, a no ka pana ana, kuhi lakou he hanu a he ea ko
loko. Ua oleloia he wai wale no ko loko o ka puuwai,
nolaila kona inoa; malia paha ua kapaia he *puukoko*, ina
ua ike pono lakou he koko ko loko o ia puu. Aole pela
ka manao o kanaka naaupo o Beritania i ka wa kahiko.
Ike pono lakou he koko maloko o na aa, a kahe no ke
moku i ka pahi. Aka, aole i maopopo ka poai ana, manao
lakou e pii ke koko i ka po mai lalo, a pau loa ke koko
iluna i ke poo paha, a i ka hele ana i ke ao emi iho la ke

Anatomia. 43

Kahi e pili ai.

Poo o ka iwi ku aoao *mawaho*.

Poo o ka iwi ku aoao ma-loko.

Kana hana.

E pelu i ka wawae.

E kokua i ke pelu ana.

Kekahi o na io malalo o ke kuli.

Kahi e pili ai	Kana hana
Ua hui pu laua i ke kaula hookahi a pili i ke kuekue.	E huki ai ke kuekue iluna, a me na manamana wawae ilalo.
Iwi kuekue kokoke i ka mea maluna.	E kokua iki i na oloolo, a e huki i ke aa malalo.
Maluna pono o ka puupuuwawae.	E hoala ai i ke kapuwai.
Iwi makia waena a me ka iwi waapa.	E huki ai i ke kapuwai iloko.
Iwi peahi o ka manamana nui.	E pelu i ka manamana nui ilalo.
Iwi peahi o ka manamana iki.	E huki i ka aoao mawaho o ke kapuwai iluna.

koko ilalo ma na wawae, nolaila ake ke kanaka e moe, no ka pau ana o ke koko o kona poo, a moe iho la huli hou ke koko a pii i ke poo, i kona wahi mamua. Oia ka mea e maha ai ke kanaka ma ka hiemoe ana, i ko lakou manao.

I ka wa kahiko, kaha kekahi poe i ke kupapau a nana aku i ka puuwai, mawaena o na aoao elua o ke ake mama, manao koke iho la lakou he mea wela loa ka puuwai, a nolaila i hoonohoia ia mawaena o na upa makani huihui, i mea e maalili ai. Manao hoi lakou o ka pana ana, oia ka lele ana o ka wai ma ka puuwai wela, oia ka mea e pana ai na aalele, o ka lele ana o ke koko, a me ka makani, a me ka ea, a me ka wela maloko. Ua hala nae ia manawa lapuwale, no ka naauao o kekahi kanaka o Beritania.

I ka makahiki o ka Haku 1620, pai iho la o Hareve i kekahi palapala e hoike ai i kona manao, no ka holo ana o ke koko a puni, maloko o ke kino. Hoike mai la oia peneia.

44   *Anatomia.*

O ka puuwai ke kumu o ke koko, a i ka upa ana o ke-kahi aoao, holo ke koko maloko o ke ake mama, a mana-mana malaila, a pilipu me na manamana makalii o ke kani ai e upa ana i ka makani; malaila i ano hou ia ke koko, a lilo ka mea eleele i ulaula, a hoi hou mai ma na aa liilii i huiia i eha aa, ua kapaia *aakoko ake mama.* Komo iho la keia koko hou a maikai ma ka *pepeiao hema* o ka puuwai, upa koke iho la ia, a komo ke koko iloko o ka *opu hema;* upa ka opu hema, a holo ke koko iloko o ke *aa lapuu,* a malaila aku ma na aalele e manamana aku ai ma ke kino a puni. Makalii loa na manamana, aole i ike maka ia, alaila huli hou ke koko ma na *aakoko* a kahe malie mai a hiki i ka pepei-ao akau o ka puuwai, maluna mai kekahi, a mai lalo mai kekahi. He koko eleele keia, a komo iloko o ka pepeiao, a kahe ke koko maloko o ka opu akau, upa iho la ia a holo hou ke koko ma ke ake mama. Pela ka hoike ana mai o Hareve, aole nae i apoia e na kanaka naauao ia ma-nawa, hoole kekahi poe me ka manao lokoino ia ia, aka, mai ia manawa mai, elua haneri makahiki a keu, ua kau-lana ia mea, o heluia o Hareve me ka poe akamai.

NO KA PUUWAI.

Ina e makemake ka haumana e ao pono i ka puuwai, e pono ia ia ke kii aku i ko ke kao paha, a i ole, i ko ka puaa paha a nana pono, no ka mea, ua like ia me ko ke kanaka.

E malama pono i ke oki ana o pokole na aa, a i nana pono ia a maopopo na mea mawaho alaila kaha. E nana oe i kahi e opu ana ma kekahi aoao, a kaha mai ka pepeiao a hala ilalo, alaila e kaha i ka lua o na opu e like me ia, a e kaka pono i ka wai a ua makaukau.

E nana i keia mau mea ma ka puuwai.

Aakoko e iho ana,
Aakoko e pii ana,
Pepeiao akau,
Opu akau,
Aalele ake mama,

Analomia. 45

Pepeiao hema,
Opu hema,
Aalele lapuu,
Aalele pokole,*
Aalele iwilei hema,
Aalele oa hema,
Aalele puuwai,
Aakoko puuwai.

E nana oe i na aoao o na opu au i kaha iho nei, a o na aoao manoanoa oia kahi o ka opu hema, a o na aoao lahilahi iki oia ko ka opu akau.

E o aku ka lima ma ka opu akau a komo i ka pepeiao akau, a malaila aku iloko o ke aakoko nui, ma ka hui ana o ke aakoko e iho ana, a me ke aakoko e pii ana, a e loaa ia oe he akea, ua lahilahi kona mau aoao, a pili uuku paha ka waha no ka oluolu ana. Mai haohao oe ke loaa ole keia aa; malama paha ua moku i ka pahi, a moku pu me ka aoao o ka pepeiao akau. E imi oe i kahi puka iki, kahi e komo mai ai ke aakoko puuwai. E hooo i ka lima ma kekahi aoao o ka opu akau, a e haha i ka puka ana aku, o ke aalele ake mama.

E haha oe maloko o ka pepeiao hema, a loaa i na puka eha o na aakoko, e komo ana mai, mai ke ake mama. E haha hoi ka lima maloko o ka opu hema, a loaa i ka puka o ke aalele lapuu. Oia na aa o ka puuwai, ewalu lakou.

NA PANI O KA PUUWAI.

E nana oe i na pani ekolu ma ke kumu o ke aalele lapuu, he aapu paha ke ano, nolaila i kapaia lakou na *pani aapu.* Aia hoi kekahi mau pani aapu ma ke kumu o ke aalele ake mama, ua like me ko ke aalele lapuu. O ka hana o keia mau pani ua like me ka ka haku o ka pauma.

E nana hou maloko o ka opu akau, he mau io huki e waiho ana, a me na kaula makalii he nui wale, e pili ana na kaula i na olona palahalaha huina kolu ekolu, a pili na

---

*Oia ke hoomanamanaia i elua, o ke aalele oa a akau a me ke aalele iwilei akau.

olona ma ke kumu i palena mawaena o ka opu, a me ka pepeiao. A ina e loaa ia oe eha olona e manao oe ua moku kekahi i elua ma ke kaha ana. E hookomo i ko manamanalima malalo o na kaula a hala loa malalo o kekahi olona, alaila e hoopili na aoao i kahaia a hapai i ke olona, e akaka ai i ke pani o ia mau olona. Ua kapaia keia mau pani *pani huina kolu.* Elua pani ma ka pepeiao hema, aka, ua like pu ka hana a me ka inoa me ko ka pepeiao akau. O na io ka mea e huki ai i na olona i pono lea ke pani ana.

E nana oe i kahi i kahaia i ka pahi, a ike pono i ke ano o ka puuwai, he io huki, aka, a le i pololei na maawe io ua hihi nui ia lakou. Oia ka mea e hiki ai i ka puuwai ke upa ikaika aku.

A pau keia mau mea i ka ikeia, e noonoo pono oe i ka holo ana o ke koko ma ka puuwai a me ka poai ana a puni ke kino.

I ka iho ana mai o ke koko eleele, mai ke poo, a me na lima mai, a i ka pii ana hoi mai na wawae, a me ka opu mai, a me ka hoi ana mai o kona koko iho, mai ka puuwai mai, ua hui pu ia ke koko ma kahi hookahi, a komo ma ka pepeiao akau o ka puuwai, a piha ka pepeiao, upa koke ia, a holo ke koko maloko o ka opu akau oiai e wehe ana oia. Oia iho la ka hana a ka pepeiao akau, o ka hoopiha i ka opu akau, a no ka hapa o kana hana ua lahilahi kona mau aoao, hookahi paha iniha, elua hapa, ka holo ana o ke koko ke upa oia.

Piha ka opu akau i ke koko, upa koke ia, lele na pani huinakolu a pili pu, ua paa ka puka aole e hoi hou ke koko ma ka pepeiao, weheia na pani aapu o ke aalele ake mama, holo pololei ke koko malaila a hoomanamanaia ma ke ake. A mohala hou ka opu hema, pili na pani aapu a paa, i hoi ole mai ke koko. Oia ka hana o ka opu akau, hookahi paha kapuwai ka holo ana o ke koko ia ia, elua paha, nolaila aole e nui kona kino me ko ka opu hema. Hana kike ka pepeiao a me ka opu, aole e kali kekahi a pau ka hana a kona hoa, aole hoi e hoolalelale.

Anatomia.   47 *

Ua like ka hana ana a ka aoao hema, me ko ka aoao akau o ka puuwai. Holo mai ke koko ulaula mai ke ake mama mai, a komo i ka pepeiao hema, upa koke oia a kipaku koke aku i ke koko, maloko o ka opu hema. O ke komo ana o ke koko, ka mea e hana ai ka opu hema, he hana nui kana, e upa i ke koko a holo aku ma ke aalele lapuu a hiki aku ma na wahi a pau loa. I kona upa ana, lele na pani aapu a pani i ka puka e komo mai ai ke koko, i puka ole aku ilaila, a i ka wehe ana o ka opu hema, aole e hoi hou mai ke koko o ke aalele lapuu, no ka mea, ua paa i na pani aapu.

Eia kekahi mea, e hana pu na pepeiao, a me na opu. E haha oe i ka pana ma ka pulima, oia ka lele ana mai o ke koko, no ka upa ana o ka opu hema. A i ka wa e hoomaha ai, oia ka wa e upa ai na pepeiao.

O ke aalele lapuu kekahi mea upa, e holo ai ke koko, pela na aalele a pau, upa no lakou e kokua ai i ka puuwai.

Ua manaoia he 33 pouna koko ma ke kino o ke kanaka, he 75 upa ana ma ka minute hookahi, a hookahi auneke koko e piha ai ka puuwai i ka upa hookahi ana. Elua minute a me ka hapalua ka poai ana o ke koko. He 24 poai ana i ka hora hookahi, a 1056 poai ana i ka la hookahi a me ka po. He ikaika loa ka opu hema i ka upa ana, i mai la kekahi poe naauao, Ua like me ke kaikai ana o na pouna he 100000! aole i akaka lea keia, aka, ua ikaika loa no.

Ua wahiia ka puuwai i ka wahi uwauwa a paa loa, aole puka e komo ai kekahi mea, he aalele kona, oia ka mea e lawe ai i koko nona, puka ia aalele ma ke kumu o ke aalele lapuu, a hoomanamanaia ma ka puuwai, ua hoihoiia keia koko maloko o ka pepeiao akau.

NO NA AALELE.

Eia kekahi mau manamana o ke aalele lapuu, o ka mua elua aalele no ka puuwai. O ka lua oia ke *aalele pokole* a manamana oia i elua, o ka *oa akau*, a me ka *iwilei akau*.

O ke kolu oia ke *oa hema*, a o ka ha ka *iwilei hema.* O ke aalele oa no ke poo ia. Ma ke aalele iwilei e hele ai ke koko ma na lima a manamana liilii malaila. O kekahi manamana ma ka pulima aole e nui ka io maluna, oia ka mea e hiki pono ai ke haha, e akaka ai ka pana ana o ka puuwai, e hiki hoi ke haha ma ke kauwahi o ke kino. Ina e upa wikiwiki ana ka puuwai, no ka wela paha ia, ina e wikiwiki loa, he kapalili paha ia, a ina paha ua akahele a nawaliwali, ina no e akaka ua kokoke e pau ka upa ana o ka puuwai, a kokoke ka make.

Holo ke aalele lapuu a pili ma ke kuamoo, a iho ilalo a hiki i ka paku mawaena o ka naau a me ke ake mama, alaila manamana aku ke aalele uuku no ke ake paa a me ke aalele no na naau. A hiki ke aalele lapuu ma ka ha o na iwi puhaka ma ka piko a maloko aku, ua puunaueia i elua, a hele kekahi ma ka wawae akau, a me kekahi ma ka wawae hema. Aole okana mai o ka nui loa o na manamana o na aalele, aka, ina e manao kekahi e ao pono ia lakou e pono ia ia ke kaha ma ke kupapau a nana pono. Ina e haha oe ma ko kino a loaa ka pana koko, e pono ke manao aia kahi aalele. Oia no ka pana ana ma na pepeiao, a ma ke poo. Oia hoi ka mea e hula ai maloko o ka opu. E akaka ia mea ma ka opu hakahaka, a nolaila kuhi hewa kekahi he mai ia. He mea nui ka ike i na aalele i ke kahuna lapaau no ka mea ina e oki oia i kekahi mai, aole e pono ke kaha naaupo, o moku hewa ke aa; aole e hiki ke hoopaa, a ina e mokuia ke aalele, ua ike pono ka mea akamai i kahi e hikii ai a paa ke koko.

NA AAKOKO.

Ma ka pau ana o na aalele liilii, malaila ke kumu o na aakoko. He mea mau ia lakou ke huipu na mea liilii i mea nui aole e manamana aku. He lahilahi ke aakoko a he akaka ma ke koko eleele maloko ke nana ma kahi uuku o ka io. He mau pani ko loko o na aakoko, oia ka

Anatomia.   49

mea e hoi ole ai ke koko mahope. Ina e mokuia ke aakoko e hiki no ke hoopili a paa ke koko, aole e huhu loa
e like me ke aalele; aole e kahe nui ke koko o ke aakoko, ke kaha uuku ia; aia i pani ia mawaena o kahi i kahaia
a me ka puuwai alaila kahe. Hele pu na aakoko me na
aalele. Mawaho kekahi malalo iho o ka ili, aole aalele
malaila no ka mea e pono ole ia mea ma kahi e moku
pinepine ia.

NO NA AALOLO.

O ke poo ke kumu o ka manao, a me ka noonoo, a ua
manaoia malaila kahi e noho ai ka uhane. O ka lolo ka
mea maloko o ke poo, ua wahiia i na aa laulau elua. Ua
hoikeia na manamana 9 o ka lolo ma ka olelo no ka iwi
opeapea, a he manamana nui ma ka puka kuamoo o ka
iwi o hope; malaila e hele ai ka lolo a puni ke kino, he
mea nui i ke aalolo ke hele pu me ke aalele, a me ke aakoko, ma kahi malu, mawaena o na io. Me he kaula
keokeo la ke aalolo, aohe puka maloko, a o kana hana oia
ka ike, a e halihali i ka ike i ka lolo. E like me ke kanaka lawaia e noho malie ana ma ka waa, a kuu ilalo i ke
aho, pela keia. Ina e lalau ka ia i ka makau ua ike koke ke kanaka, ua pii mai ka ike ia ia ma ke aho, a ina ua
moku ke aho, ina ua ike ole ke kanaka i ka lalau ana o
ka ia. Noho malie ka uhane ma ka lolo a hele na kaula
aalolo he kinikini mai ka lolo aku i na wahi a pau o ka
ili: ina e pa aku kekahi mea ma ka ili, ua ike koke ke
kanaka, ua pii mai ka ike ma ke aalolo: a hiki mai i ka
lolo a ina ua moku ke aalolo, aole loa e ike ke kanaka ke
hoopa aku kekahi mea ia ia, ua maeele.

Ua ike paha na kanaka a pau, i ka maeele o ka uha, ke
noho kapakahi a liuliu. No ka pilikia o ke aalolo ka maeele, a ina i hikiiia i ke kaula, maeele no; no ka mea, aole
e hiki i ka ike ke pii ma kahi pilikia. Oia ke ano o ka
mai lolo, ua pilikia na aalolo; no ka pehu paha o kekahi
manawa, a no ka hu hewa ana o ke koko i kekahi manawa, ka mea e pilikia ai.

5

50   *Anatomia.*

Ua hoonohoia ka uhane maloko o ke kino i haku, e alii ana maluna. O ka lolo kona noho alii, a o na aalolo kona mau elele hoounauna, a i ole ia, o na aalele ka mau alanui kahi e hiki ai na elele ke holo. Eia wau ke palapala nei, e waiho ana ko'u lima hema ma ka papa, lele mai la ka nalo a aki ma kuu kuli, pii koke iho la ka ike ma na aalolo a hiki ma ke poo. Alaila manao iho la au e kipaku, holo koke aku la ka manao ma na aalolo a hiki aku i na io, olelo aku la ia lakou e huki, hana koke iho la lakou, a lawe i ka lima ilalo i ke kuli, e kahili aku i ua mea kolohe la. Meneia na hana a pau, holo mai ka ike a holo aku ma na aalele, aole nae i manao ke kanaka ma ia mea. Ma na maka mai ka nui o ka ike, nana aku ka maka a lawelawe na lala; pela no ka pepeiao. Kahea mai la paha kekahi ia oe, lohe koke ka pepeiao, manao koke iho la oe e hele ilaila, huki koke ka *io alaea* a me na io a pau, o ka hele no ia o na wawae. Pela ka honi ana, a me ka hoao ana o ka waha, he mau ike okoa keia, ma na aalolo nae ka holoholo ana a me ka hoomaopopo ana.

O ka mea a kakou e kapa ai, *o ka naau* aia kona wahi e noho ai ma ke poo, aole ina ka opu; ua like pu ka naau me ka uhane: aka, ina i manao kekahi ua okoa, o ka naau ka hana a o ka uhane ka mea nana i hana. Pela ka manao, no ka uhane mai ia. A hiki ka manawa e kii mai ai ke Akua i ka uhane, a lawe aku, alaila pau ka hana, pau ka hanu ana o ke ake mama, pau ka upa ana o ka puuwai a me ka huki ana o na io: pili na maka, kuli na pepeiao, moe malie ke kanaka he kupapau, a lilo koke i ka pala kahuki ia. Ua hala ka uhane i ke Akua, a i ka ukuia e like me kana hana.

Aole e mau ke kaawale ana o ka uhane a me ke kino. E hui hou ia laua. E hooala hou ia ke kupapau mai ka lepo mai, a mai ka moana mai, a mai kona wahi e helelei ai, a komo ka uhane ia ia; alaila e hanaia ka mea i oleloia'i ma ka Mataio, Mokuna 25; pauku 31, a hiki i ka pau ana o ka mokuna.

Anatomia.   51

NO KA OPU.

Alua *kea* i ka olelo ana; o ke *kea paa* a me ke *kea ha-kahaka.* O ke *ake mama*, a me ka *puuwai*, oia na mea maloko o ke kea paa; a o ke *ake paa*, a me ka *opu*, a me ke *ake niau*, a me na *puupaa*, a me ke *koana mimi*, oia ke-kahi mau mea maloko o ke kea hakahaka.

O ka *paku* mawaena o na kea, he io huki ia, ua pili ma na iwi aoao olalo, a me ke kuamoo, a me ka iwi umauma. He io keia no ka hanu ana, a i kona huki ana ua like me ka mea omo; a huki ilalo ke ake mama, alaila komo mai ka makani ma ka ihu, e pani ai i ka hakahaka. O ka lele ana o ka oili, a me ke kapalili ana o ka houpo, oia paha ka eeke ana o keia paku o na kea.

O ke *ake paa* oia ma ka aoao akau, malalo ae o na aoao a hiki i ka houpo. O ke *au* kana mea e hana'i noloko mai o ke koko. I ka hoi ana mai o ke koko eleele, mai na naau mai, a hele i ka puuwai, komo na aakoko maloko o ke akepaa a ua hoomanamana hou ia lakou malaila, i hoo-kaawaleia ke au noloko mai o ua koko eleele la. Alaila hui pu ia na aakoko i hookahi, a pii aku, a komo iloko o ke *aakoko e pii ana.* Ua waihoia ke au maloko o kona aa, a hiki i ka manawa e ai ai ke kanaka i ka ai, kahe aku la ke au, a komo iloko o ka opu e huiia me ka ai. Aole i akaka lea ke kuleana o ke au malaila: ua manaoia, oia ka mea e hookaawale ai ka mea maikai o ka ai, a koe ka mea ino, a me ke okaoka.

Aia ma ka aoao hema ka *opu.* Oia ka laulau no ka ai, he lahilahi, a he nui ke koko maloko o na aa mawaho ona. O ka hana, oia ka hoonapele i ka ai.

O ke *ake niau*, he ake loloa ia e pili ana mawaho o ka opu; aole i akaka kana hana. Olelo kekahi poe he wai-hona koko no ka opu, no ka nui o ke koko maloko ona, aole nae i ike pono ia.

Alua ano o na *naau*, o ka mea nui a me ka mea liilii. Ua uhiia lakou a pau e ka *makaupena.* Aia ka mua o na naau liilii, ma ka pau ana o ka opu. Hookahi kapuwai

kona loihi, nolaila i kapaia *naau kapuwai.* Ma keia naau
e komo ai ka nuku o ke au. Mai ka naau kapuwai a
hiki i ka naau nui, eha anana ka loa o na naau liilii, a he
hookahi paha iniha ka nui ke anaia mai kekahi aoao a i
kekahi aoao. Ua poai ka naau liilii a anapuu a puni ka
piko, alaila komo iloko o ka naau nui o *kauha* kona inoa,
aole e komo kekahi piko o ka naau iloko o kekahi e like
me ka naau kapuwai; ua komo huina ha maluna aku o ke
poo o kauha. Elima kapuwai ka loa o kauha, aia kona poo
ma ka hena akau; pii mai la ia mai ka puupaa akau, a huli
ae malalo iho o ke akepaa, a mawaho o na naau *liilii*, a hiki i
ka aoao hema malalo iki ae o ka opu, alaila hoi ilalo a
hele kekee, a hiki i ka iwi kikala, malaila e iho ai mawaena konu a puka aku mawaho.

Eia ke ano o ka hele ana o ka ai mai luna a lalo. Komo ka ai iloko o ka waha, e nauia e na niho a wali, a huipuia me ka wale o ka waha; oia kekahi mea e hooheehee
ai, alaila mai iho la; hele ka ai maluna o ke alelo, a maluna hoi o ka puka o ke kaniai, poi mai la ke kileo a
paa ka puka, i komo ole ka ai ma ke kaniai, iho aku la
ka mana ai a komo iloko o ka opu; malaila e huiia'i me ka
wai o ka opu, he wai pahee a he ikaika hoi i ka hooheenee. Oia, a me ke kuha i moniia mamua, a me ka mahana, a me ka mahola ana o ka opu, ka mau mea e lilo
koke ai ka ai i behee, a komo iloko o ka naau kapuwai.
Ua omoia kekahi o keia mea heehee i ka wa e noho ana
maloko o ka opu, a ma ka naau kapuwai, omoia no, a pela e omoia a hala na anana elima o na naau, a pau ka
momona o ka ai, a koe wale no ka mea ino. He kinikini
na *aaomo* e hookomo ana ko lakou waha ma na naau a
pau, he liilii me he hulu puaa la ka nui, a ua piha lakou i
ka ai heehee, ua like me ka waiu kona ano. Huiia na
aaomo i hookahi ma ka aoao hema o ke kuamoo, ua like
kona nui me he hulu nene la, he keekee nae ka waiho
ana. Pii ka wai momona ma keia aa a hiki ma ka ai,
alaila komo iloko o ke aakoko o ka lima hema, a holopu
me ke koko a hiki i ka puuwai ,a malaila aku, a hiki i na

Anatomia.   59

Wahi a pau, e lilo ai i io, a i iwi, a i momona, a i na mea
a pau loa e ikaika ai ke kino.   He holo mau keia, nolaila,
aole e pono ke kanaka ke noho wale, aole e ai i ka ai.   O
ka ai pinepine ka pono, i ekolu paha ai ana i ka la hookahi, aka, aole e pono ke hooluhi hewa i ka opu a hoohana
nui ia ia i ka ai nui loa, o kaumaha a awaawa ka ai maloko o ka opu.   He kumu ia o ka *haoa* a me ke nahu, a
me ka wela o ka opu, a me ka hoopailua, a me ka luai, i
pau ka mea e hiki ole ai ia ia ke hana i ke kiolaia'ku, a
haalele.   Eia kekahi hewa nui o ke puhi baka, o ke kuha
wale ia'ku o ka wale o ka waha, ka mea e pono ke moniia
i mea e hooheehee ai i ka ai; a ina paha ua moniia, ina
no ua awaawa i ka uwahi baka.   O ke puhi baka ka mea
e nawaliwali ai ka opu, i hiki ole ai ia ia ke hana i ka ai
e pono ai ke kanaka.   O ka hana maoli o ke kino kekahi
mea e pono ai; oia ka mea e emi ai ke kino, a o ka ai ka
mea emi ai.   E like paha me ka mahinaai; o ka wai ka
ka mea e ulu nui ai ka ai, a o ka la ka mea e pau ai ka
wai; aka, ina he ua wale no, aole he la kekahi, ina ua
pono ole ka ai, ua loliloli.   Pela ka *hana* e pono ai ke kanaka.   Nolaila, ina aole e hana kekahi aole ia e pono ke ai.
    E nana ma ke Kauoha Hou, ma ka palapala lua a Paulo
i ko Teselonike, Mokuna 3: Pauku 10, a heluhelu.
    Aia na PUUPAA ma ke kuamoo, maloko o ke konahua,
ma ka akau kekahi ma ka hema kekahi, a maluna iki ae
o na iwi papakole.   O ka laua oihana, oia ka hookaawale
i ka mimi noloko mai o ke koko, nolaila holo nui ke koko
malaila, ma ke aalele mimi, he manamana o ke aalele
lapuu.   Pakahi ka auwai loihi no laua e kahe ai ka mimi a
komo ma ka aoao malalo o ke koana mimi: he umi iniha ka loa o keia auwai.   He wai ka mimi, he paakai kekahi mea maloko, a me ka puna, a me ia mea aku, ia mea
aku; he umikumamakahi mau mea maloko o ka wai
mimi, a nui na mea e hele ai mailoko aku o ke kino ma ka
mimi ana.   A i kekahi manawa e huiia na paakai a me
ka puna, a nui ka haku, aole e hiki ke puka aku, ulu ia i
pohaku nui no ka hui mau ana mai o ka puna maloko o
    5*

ka mimi. O ke kaa ana o ua pohaku la maloko o ke
koana mimi, he mea eha loa ia a make loa ke kanaka i ka
eha. Nolaila kaha ka poe ike ma ia hana, a komo i loko
o ke koana mimi, houia ka upa maloko, lalau ia ka pohaku, a unuhiia mai la.

Ua nui na wai i koe, noloko mai o ke koko. O ka *hou*
kekahi mea nui noloko mai o na manamana aalele makalii ma ka ili, a no ka makalii o lakou puka ka wai wale no
aole e hiki aku ke koko ulaula. Malaila kekahi kumu o
ka mai, no ka mea i ka wa e pa mai ai ka makani huihui,
a o ka wai anu paha, pili koke na waha a pau o keia mau
aa; hooikaika iho la ka puuwai i kana hana e puka aku ai
ka wai, aole e hiki, wela mai la ke kino, inoino maloko o
ka opu, no ka wela; a no ka holo ikaika paha o ke koko
ma ke ake paa, nui ke au i hanaia, oia no ka lena. A o
ka puholoholo, kekahi mea e pono ai, a o ka laau naha
kekahi i puka ka wai malaila. He paakai kekahi maloko
o ka hou, a he puna no kekahi. O ka *upe* kekahi wai ua
hanaia e na aalele o ka ihu. O ka *wale* o ka waha, na
na anoano ia e hana, aia malalo o ke elelo kekahi a ma
na hookuina iwi a lalo kekahi a ma kahi e kekahi.

O KA HOOMAOPOPO ANA I NA KII.

E nana oe i ka hua palapala a i ka hua helu paha ma
keia palapala, a o ka hua like ma ke kii oia ka mea i hoakaka ia.

KII I.

Ua hooiliiliia'i na iwi a pau o ke kanaka a hookuiia'i a
pili pono kekaki i kekahi. Eia na iwi i ikeia ma ke alo,
o ka hua palapala he kuhi ia i ka hua e like pu ana ma
ke kii.

O NA IWI O KE POO.

a, Iwi lae.	h,h, Iwi papalina.
e, Iwi hua.	k, Iwi a luna.
i, Iwi maha.	l, Iwi a lalo.
o, Iwi opeapea.	m, Iwi ai.
u, Iwi ihu.	

Anatomia.   55

O NA IWI O KE KINO.

a, Iwi kua he 12.
e, Iwi puhaka he 5.
i,i, Iwi umauma.
o, Iwi aoao oluna he 7.

u,u,u, Iwi aoao lalo he 5.
h, Iwi ka.
k,k, Iwi papakole.
l, Iwi puukole.
m,m, Iwi lemu.

O NA IWI O KA LALA O LUNA.

a,a, Iwi lei.
e,e, Iwi hoehoe.
i,i, Iwi uluna.
o,o, Iwi kano.

u,u, Iwi kubita.
h,h, Iwi pulima.
k,k, Iwi manamanalima.

O NA IWI O KA LALA OLALO.

a,a, Iwi hilo.
e,e, Huamoa
i,i, Iwi kuapoi.
o,o, Iwi ku.

u,u, Iwi pili.
h,h, Iwi kuekue.
k,k, Iwi manamanawawae.

KII II.

Ma keia kii ua hoohuliia'i ke kanaka a ikea mai na iwi o ke kua.

O NA IWI O KE POO.

a,a, Iwi hua.
e, Iwi hope.
i, Iwi maha.

o, Iwi papalina.
u, Iwi a lalo.

O NA IWI O KE KINO.

a, Iwi ai.
e, Iwi kua.
i, Iwi puhaka.

o,o, Iwi papakole.
u, Iwi kikala.
h, Iwi okole.

O NA IWI O KA LALA OLUNA.

a,a, Iwi lei.
e,e, Iwi hoehoe.
i,i, Iwi uluna.
o,o, Iwi kano.

u,u, Iwi kubita.
h,h, Iwi pulima.
k,k, Iwi manamanalima.

O NA IWI O KA LALA OLALO.

a,a, Iwi hilo.
e,e, Iwi ku.
i,i, Iwi pili.

o,o, Iwi kuekue.
u,u, Iwi puupuuwawae.
h,h, Iwi manamanawawae

36   *Anatomia.*

KII III.

3
Iwi LAE.
a,a, Hakahaka.
e,e, Makalua.
i,i, Oi ihu
o, Lapa io maha.
u,u, Lihi kuemaka.

5
Piko o ke poo.
u, Iwi lei.
e,e, Iwi hua.
i. Iwi hope.
1,1, Hoai manawa.
2,2, Hoai kaupaku.
3,3, Hoai kala.
4,4. Hoai maha.
o, Manawa hope.
u, Manawa mua.

4
Iwi MAHA.
a, Hapa unahi.
e, Oi apo.
i, Kumu pepeiao.
o, Oi kui.
u, Puka pepeiao mawaho.

6
Iwi ELELO.

7
NA IO O KA PEPEIAO.
1, Hamare.
2, Kua.
3, Keehi.
4, Keehi ua huliia ilalo.
5, Iwi hoehoe.

8
Iwi OPEAPEA.
1,1, Eheu nui ma ka maha.
2,2, Eheu iki.
3,3,3,3, Na wawae.

KII IV.

7
Ke kuamoo.
1,2,3,4,5,6, He mau aalolo
e puka mai ana mawaena o
ke kuamoo.
7. Pauku o ka naau liilii.
8, Iwi okole.
9,9, Na puupaa.
10, Akepaa.
11, Opu.

8
He iwi ai.
a, Kona kino.
e, Ka oi waena ua hoomanamanaia.
i, Wahi e pili ai me kekahi
w .
o,o, Oi aoao.
u, Puka aalolo kuamoo.

9
Iwi UMAUMA.
a,a, Kahi e pili ai me ka
iwi lei.
e,e, Kahi o ka iwi aoao mua.
i, Kahi o ke kaniai

10
Iwi PUHAKA.
a. Kona kino.
e, Oi waena.
i,i, Kahi e hui ai me kekahi
iwi.

Anatomia. 57

o,o,o, Ma keia mau wahi ka *o,o,* Oi aoao.
pili ana o na iwi aoao.
u, Kahi e pili ai ka pilali
iwi umauma.

KII V.

11	12
HOOKUINA O KA HUAMOA.	HOEHOE.

1, Iwi papakole.	1, Iwi lei.
2, Lua no ka huamoa.	2, Iwi umauma.
3, Iwi hilo.	3, Iwi hoehoe.
4, Huamoa.	4, Iwi uluna.
5, Kaula olona.	

13	14
KUEKUELIMA.	PULIMA MALOKO.

1,1, Iwi kano.	1, Iwi kubita.
2,2, Iwi kubita.	2, Iwi kano.
3,3, Iwi uluna.	

15	16
PULIMA MALOKO.	PEAHILIMA.

1, Iwi waapa.	1, Lima kuhi.
2, Iwi mahina.	2, Lima loihi.
3, Iwi makia.	3, Lima komo.
4, Iwi poepoe.	4, Lima iki.
5, Iwi ahalike.	
6, Iwi ewaewa.	
7, Iwi nui.	
8, Iwi lou.	

KII VI.

21	22
PUUPUUWAWAE.	KAPUUWAI.

1,1,1, Iwi ku.	1, Iwi ami.
2,2,2, Iwi pili.	2, Iwi kuekue.
3,3,3, Na olona.	3, Iwi ipuka.
	4, Iwi ahalike.
	5, Iwi makia kolu.
	6, Iwi makia lua.
	7, Iwi makia mua.

23	24
Iwi manamanawawae.	Iwi manamanawawae nui.

58   *Anatomia.*

KII VII.

25   26

Kekuli.   HE LIMA UA PAA I NA OLONA.

1, Iwi kano.
2, Iwi kubita.

27

He wawae ua paa i na olona.

KII VIII.

29   30

NA IO O KA MAKA.

1, Ohope lae.	1, Ohopelae.
2, Pukupukuemaka.	2, Puhi.
3, Poailihilihi.	3, Hooewanuku mua.
4, Mimino.	4, Hooewanuku waena.
5, Hooewanuku mua.	5, Hooewanuku hope.
6, Hooewanuku waena	6, Alawa.
7, Hoopinanalehelehe luna.	7, Haku hana wale no ka
8, Puhi.	waha.
9, Poaiwaha.	
10,10, Pelulehelehe lalo.	

KII IX.

31   32

1, Alawa.	1, Kulanaaoao mawaho.
2, Oakaloihi.	2, Kulanaaoao maloko.
3, Kaniai.	3, Kupono.
4, Iwilei.	4, Kuoi.
	5,5, Iliwai.
	6,6, Kaha keokeo.

KII X.

33   34

1, Pani oloko.	1, Eeke.
2, Papakole maloko.	2, Kau nui.
3, Uhao nui.	3, Kau uuku.
4, Lihi iwi papakole.	4, Niho mole mua.
	5, Hio mawaho.

KII XI.

35   36

1, Kaha.	
2, Hoehoe luna.	1, Hokua.
3, Hoehoe lalo.	2, Huinaha hio kua.
4, Palahalaha kua.	3,3, Palahalaha kua.

5, Mole nui.
6, Mole uuku.
7, Kumukolu.
8, Uluna.

4, Nihomole lalo.
5, Apana.
6,7, Lemu nui.

37
1, Olapa omole.
2, Pelu peahi oloko.
3, Poho lima.
4, Pelu peahi owaho.
5, Uala.

KII XII.
1,1,1,1,1, Hokua.
2, Palahalaha kua.
3, Kaha.
4, Hoehoe lalo.
5, Kumu kolu.
6, Alawa.

KII XIII.
38
1, Olona kupec.
2, Mohala manamanalima.
3, Mohala lima iki.
39
1, Pelu manamanalima.
40
1, Olapa omole.
2, Olapa ahalike.

KII XIV.

41
1, Lemu waena.
2, Kapakahi.
3, Aalolo wawae.
4, Poolua.
5, Olona lemu.
6, He aalolo.
8, He aalele, a mawaena o laua he aakoko.
9,9, Oloolo wawae.

42
1, Hoahaaha.
2,2, Alaea.
3, Kuapoi.
4, Pololei uha.
5, Aalele.
43
O na aalele o ka ia, a me ka puuwai.
a, puuwai.

KII XV.

44
O na aa, a me na io.
1, Io Pololei ua okiia.
2, Hoahaaha.
3, Alaea.
4, Ke aalele.
5, Ke aakoko.
6, Ke aalolo.

45
1, O na aakoko.
2, Aalele.
3, Oloolowawae.
46
O na aoao elua o ka puuwai, ua hookaawaleia.

60   *Anatomia.*

KII XVI.

47 48   49
O na wawae, ua kahaia e   Kapepeiao.
ikea'i na io, a me na kaula,
1, Olona kupee.

KII XVII.

50 51   53
O na wawae.
1, Oloolo wawae.   O ka maka.
2, Libini.   1, Aalolo nana.
        52   2, Onohe akaka.
Pepeiao oloko.   3,4,5, Na wahi o ka maka.
                             6, Poniu.

KII XVIII.

54   55
O ka Puuwai.   O na manamana o ke aalele
1, Aakoko e iho ana.   oa, ua mokuia ka iwi puniu
2, Aakoko e pii ana.   e ka pahiolo e ikea mai ai ka
3, Aakoko akepaa.   lolo a me na manamana o ke
4, Aalele akemama.   aalele lolo, *a.*
5, Aakoko akemama.   1, Aalele oa.
6, Aalele lapuu.   2,3, Na io Hooewanuku i
7, Aalele pokole.   okiia i ka pahi.
8, Aalele oa hema.   4, Puhi.
9, Aalele iwilei hema.   5, Nau.
10, Opu hema.
11, Pepeiao hema.   O na pua ka mea e akaka ai
12, Pepeiao akau.   ka holo ana o ke koko malo-
X, Aakoko puuwai.   ko o na aa.

KII XIX.

56   57
O ka lolo, a me na manama-   Na naau.
na lolo i kahaia a kaawale. 1, Opu.
1, Lolo.   2, Kauha.
2, Manamana o ka 5 o na   3, Naau nui.
aalolo.   4, Naau liilii.
3, Aalolo iwi aoao.
4, Aalolo Puhaka.
5, Aalolo kikala.

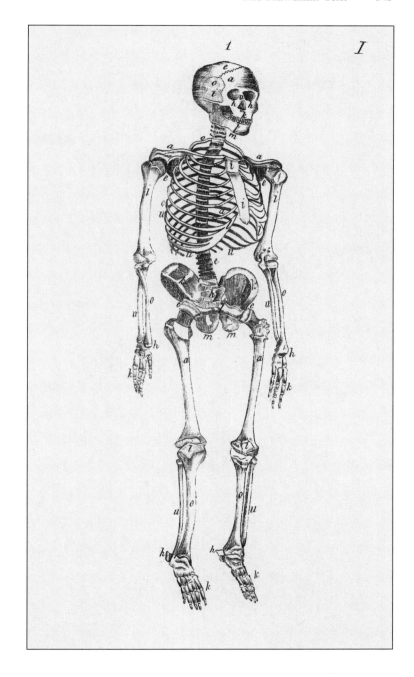

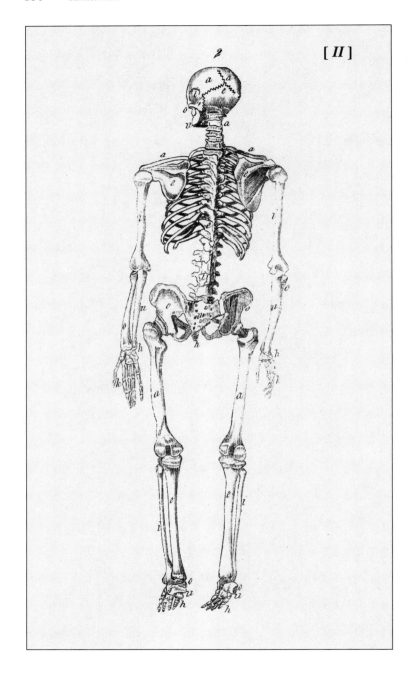

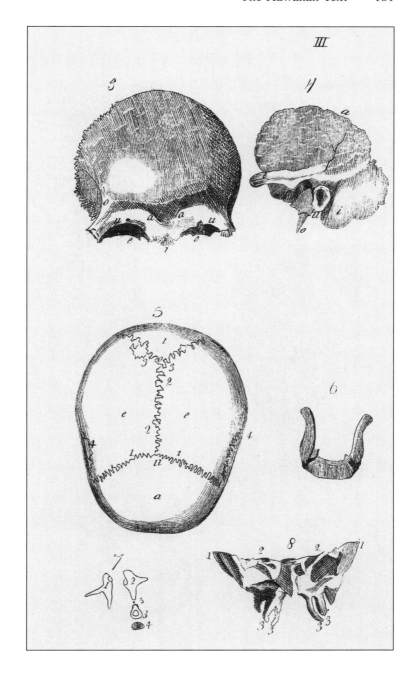

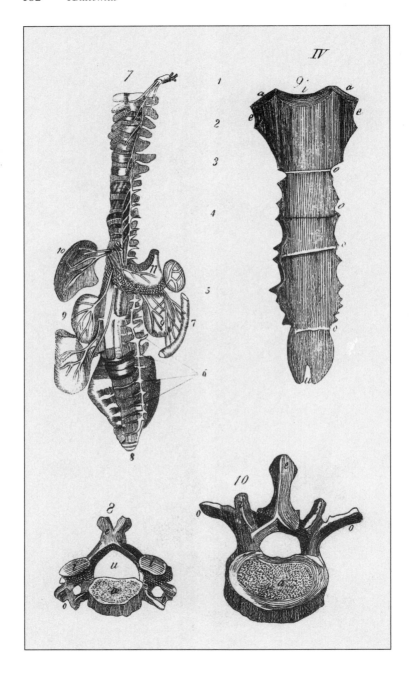

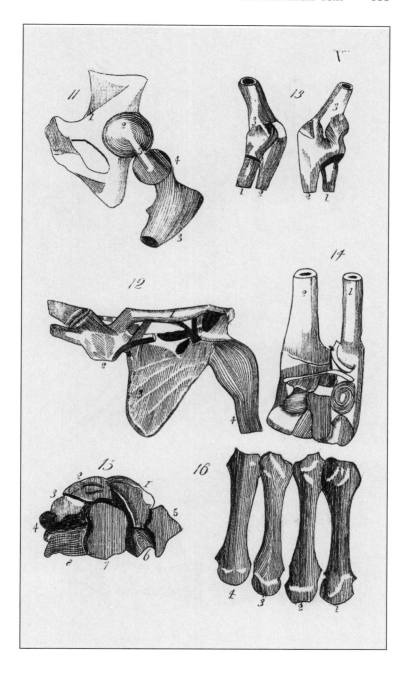

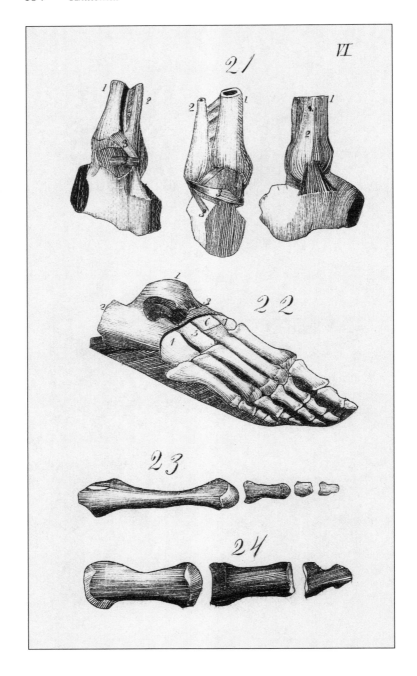

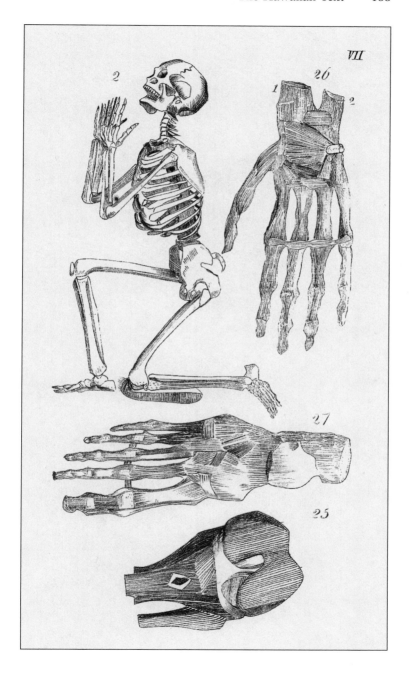

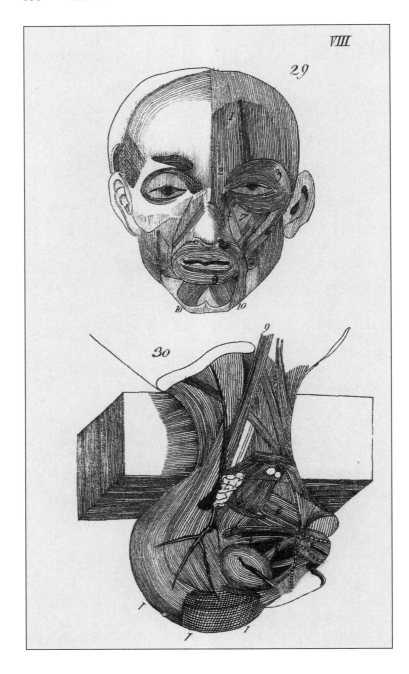

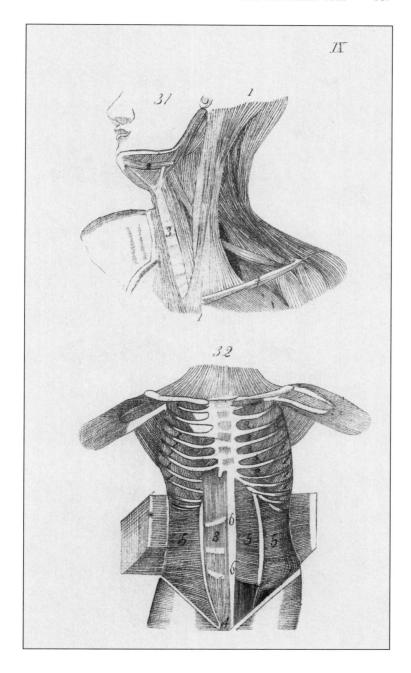

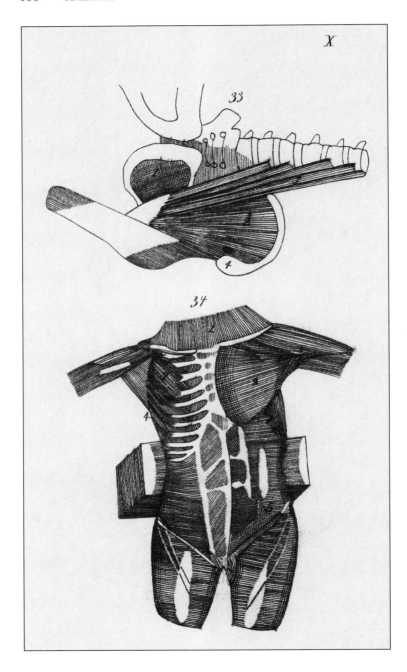

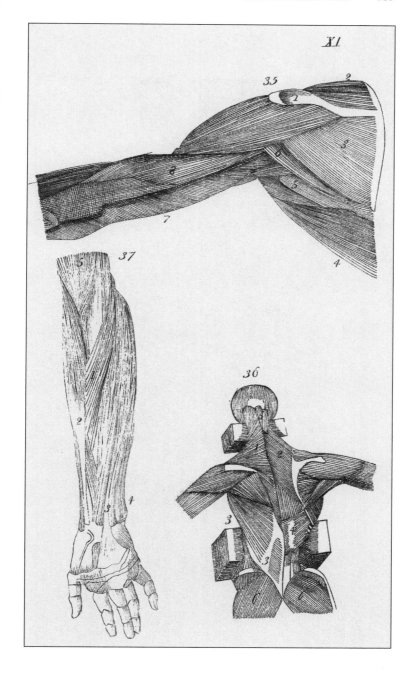

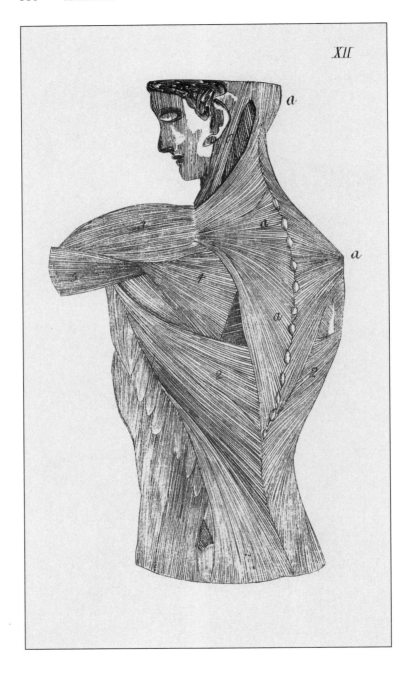

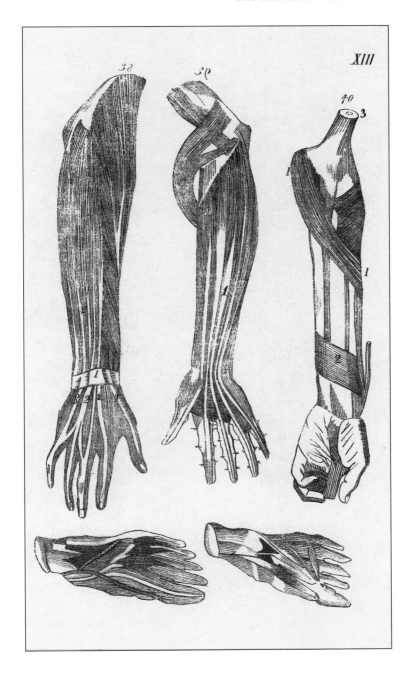

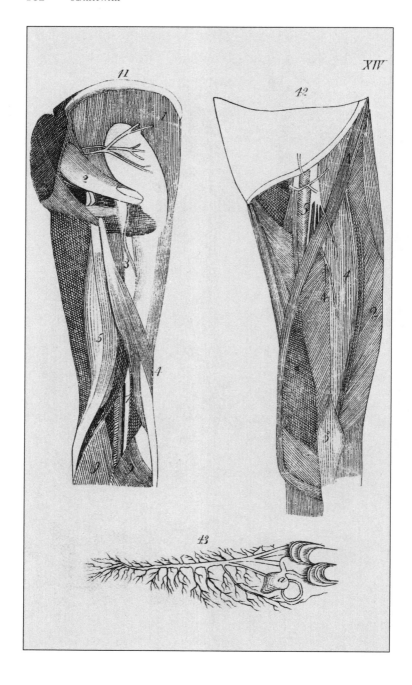

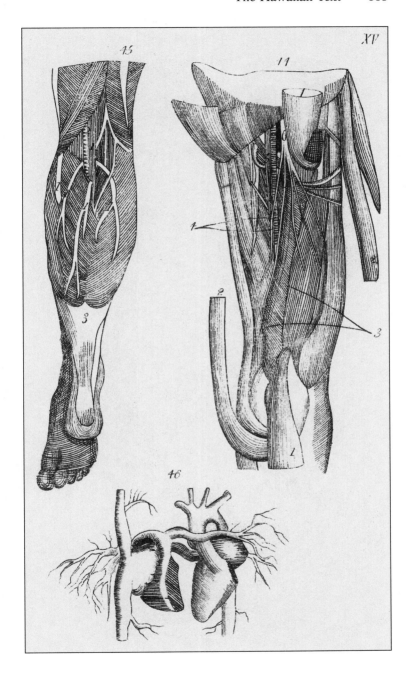

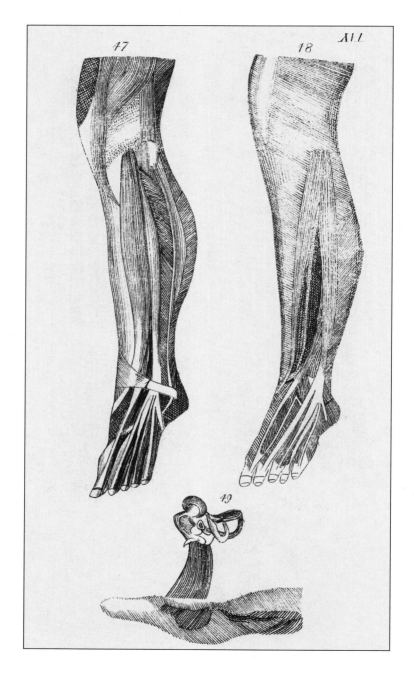

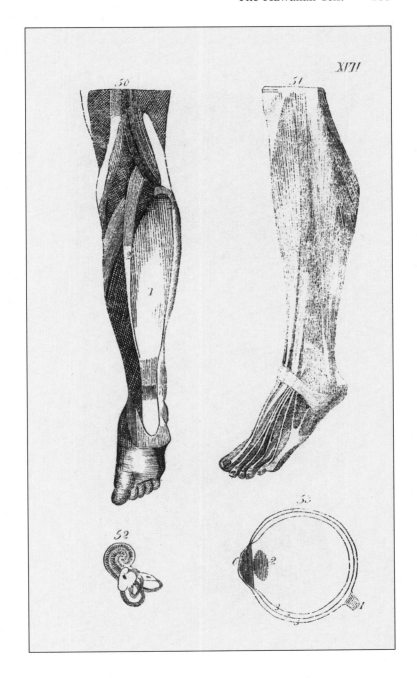

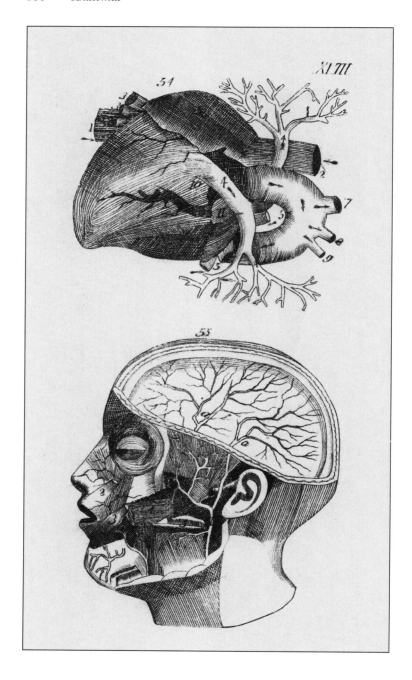

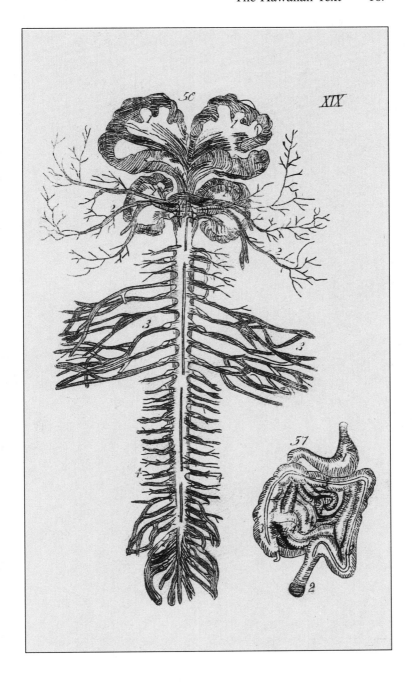

GLOSSARY 1
HAWAIIAN–ENGLISH

aa	blood vessel
aakoko	vein
aakoko ake mama	pulmonary vein
aakoko e iho ana	descending/superior vena cava
aakoko e pii ana	ascending/inferior vena cava
aakoko puuwai	coronary vein
aa lapuu	aorta
aa laulau	ligaments resembling netting
aalele	artery
aalele ake mama	pulmonary artery
aalele iwi lei akau	right subclavian artery
aalele iwi lei hema	left subclavian artery
aalele mimi	renal artery
aalele oa	carotid artery
aalele oa akau	right carotid artery
aalele oa hema	left carotid artery
aalele puuwai	coronary artery
aalolo	nerve
aalolo hoao	taste nerve
aalolo honi	olfactory nerve
aalolo kuamoo	spinal nerve
aalolo lohe	auditory nerve
aalolo nana	optic nerve
aaomo	lymphatic
ake	liver
ake mama	lung
ake niau	spleen
ake paa	liver
alelo, elelo	tongue
ami	joint
ana	antrum
anoano	salivary gland
apo	band where cheek bone and temporal bone unite

au	bile
auwae	chin
eha	pain
elua pani ma ka pepeiao hema	bicuspid valve in left auricle
haoa	heartburn
hapa oolea	petrous part
hapa unahi	squamous part
hoai	suture
hoai kala	lambdoidal suture
hoai kaupaku	sagittal suture
hoai maha	temporal suture
hoai manawa	coronal suture
hookauhua	growing state of the young in the womb
hookuina ami	hinged joint
hookuina lewa	floating joint
hoopailua	nausea
hou	perspiration
houpo	thorax
hua moa	head in the femur
huinaha	square
io	muscle
io huki	pulling muscle
io kokua	voluntary muscle
io kuokoa	involuntary muscle
iokupu	polypus
io maha	temple muscle
io nau	chewing muscle
iwi	bone
iwi ahalike	cuboides (foot); trapezium (hand)
iwi ai	cervical bone
iwi a lalo	mandible
iwi alelo (elelo)	hyoid bone
iwi a luna	maxilla
iwi ami	heel or calcaneum
iwi anoano	sesamoid bone (foot)
iwi aoao	ribs
iwi ewaewa	trapezoides (hand)
iwi hamare	mallet (ear)
iwi hilo	femur
iwi hoehoe	scapula
iwi hope	occipital bone
iwi hua	parietal bone
iwi ihu	nasal bone

iwi ipukai	naviculare (foot)
iwi ka, (puhaka)	loin bones or pelvis
iwi kanana	ethmoid bone
iwi kano	radius
iwi keehi	stapes (ear)
iwi kikala	sacrum
iwi kileo	palate bone
iwi ku	tibia
iwi kua	anvil (ear); dorsal bone
iwi kuamoo	vertebrae
iwi kuapoi	patella
iwi kubita	ulna
iwi kuekue	ankle bone or astragalus
iwi lae	frontal bone
iwi lei	clavicle
iwi lemu	buttocks bone
iwi lou	unciforme (hand)
iwi maha	temporal bone
iwi mahina	lunare (hand)
iwi makia	cuneiforme (hand)
iwi makia kolu	third or lateral cuneiforme (foot)
iwi makia lua	second or intermediate cuneiforme (foot)
iwi makia mua	first or medial cuneiforme (foot)
iwi manamanalima	finger or phalange
iwi manamanawawae	toe or phalange
iwi mua o ka ai	first cervical bone, atlas
iwi nui	magnum (hand)
iwi okole	coccyx
iwi opeapea	sphenoid bone
iwi owili	turbinated bone
iwi paku	vomer
iwi papakole	hip bone
iwi papalina	cheek or malar bone
iwi peahilima	metacarpus
iwi peahi wawae	fan-shaped bone (foot) or metatarsus
iwi pepeiao	ear bone
iwi pili	fibula
iwi poepoe	round bone (ear); orbiculare (hand)
iwi poo	head bone
iwi poohiwi	shoulder bone
iwi puhaka	loin bones, pelvis
iwi pulima	carpus
iwi puukole	pubic bone
iwi puupuuwawae	tarsus

iwi uluna	humerus
iwi umauma	sternum
iwi waapa	naviculare (hand)
iwi waimaka	lachrymal bone
kaha keokeo	white line
kahuna lapaau	physician
kani ai	trachea
kapalili	palpitation
kauha	colon
kaula	tendon
kea hakahaka	abdomen
kea paa	chest
koana mimi	urinary bladder
koko	blood
koko eleele	venous [black] blood
konahua	inside fat of man and animals
kua	back
kuamoo	spine or vertebra
kuekue	a joint
kuekue lima	elbow
kuemaka	eyebrow
kui	bicuspids; styloid process
kui nui	molars
kumu pepeiao	ear base
laau naha	cathartic medicine
lala o lalo	lower extremities
lala o luna	upper extremities
lapaau	medicine
lele	to overlap
lepe	cock's comb
lolo	brain; marrow of bone
luamaka	same as *makalua*, eye socket
luauhane	tear duct
mai	disease
mai lolo	brain disease
maka	face
makalua	eye socket, same as *luamaka*
makani,	air one breathes
maloeloe	firm
mana ami	hinge branch in mandible
manamana lima	finger
manamana makalii	bronchi
manamana nui	thumb

manamana wawae	toe
mana mua	front branch in mandible
manawa	fontanel
manawa hope	posterior fontanel
manawa mua	anterior fontanel
momona	fat
naau	intestine
naau kapuwai	duodenum
niho ai waiu	incisors
niho oo,	wisdom teeth
niho paa	permanent teeth
nuku o ke au	duct of the gall bladder
oa akau	right carotid
oa hema	left carotid
oi	projection
oi lapa	flat projection
oi nuku	noselike projection
okupe	to sprain
ole	cuspids
olona	ligament
olona palahalaha huina kolu, ekolu	three triangular flat ligaments
oolea	hard
opu	a protuberance with an enclosure, such as the heart or stomach
opu akau	right ventricle
opu hema	left ventricle
opuupuu	convex
paku mawaena oka naau a me ke ake mama	diaphragm
pala	syphilis
pana koko	pulse
pani aapu	valves
pani huinakolu	tricuspid valve
papalina	the cheek or side of a face
pepeiao	ear
pepeiao akau	right auricle
pepeiao hema	left auricle
pilali	cartilage
poholima	hollow or palm of hand
poo	head
poohiwi iki	lesser trochanter
poohiwi nui	greater trochanter

puao	womb
puhaka	pelvis
puholoholo	a perspiration produced by the steam covering over a fire; the patient sits covered with a kapa over it
puka nana	optic nerve
puka pepeiao maloko	internal ear
puka pepeiao mawaho	external ear
pulima	wrist
puna	calcium
puupaa	kidney
puupuu	protuberance
puuwai	heart
uahau, uhau	to be embedded in
uala	biceps
unahi	scaly, squamous part of the temple bone
une	lever
upoho	concave
uwauwa	tough
wai	fluid
wale o ka waha	saliva

GLOSSARY 2
MUSCLES:
HAWAIIAN–LATIN

Ahalike puhaka	Quadratus lumborum
Ahalike uha	Quadratus femoris
Alaea	Rectus femoris or Rectus cruris
Alawa	Sterno-cleido-mastoideus
Alo uha	Vastus externus
Apana	Splenius
Auwiolalo	Obliquus inferior
Auwioluna	Obliquus superior or Trochlearis
Eeke	Platysma myoides
Haikaikanuku	Depressor anguli oris
Hena	Pectinalis
Hiomaloko	Obliquus ascendens internus
Hiomawaho	Obliquus descendens externus
Hoahaaha	Sartorius
Hoalaloihi	Extensor carpi radialis longus
Hoalapokole	Extensor carpi radialis brevior
Hoehoelalo	Infraspinatus
Hoehoeluna	Supraspinatus
Hokua	Trapezius or Cucullaris
Hooala lima nui	Extensor ossis metacarpii pollicis manus
Hooala peahi	Extensor carpi ulnaris
Hooewanuku hope	Zygomaticus minor
Hooewanuku mua	Levator angulis oris
Hooewanuku waena	Zygomaticus major
Hoopinana lehelehe luna	Levator labii superioris proprius
Hoopololei lua o ka lima nui	Extensor secundi internodii
Hoopololei mua o ka lima nui	Extensor primi internodii
Huinaha hio kua	Rhomboides
Iliwai	Transversalis abdominis

Iwilei	Subscapularis
Kaakaamaka	Levator palpebrae superioris
Kaha	Deltoid
Kahalua	Coraco brachialis
Kahela loihi	Adductor longis femoris
Kahela nui	Adductor magnus femoris
Kahela pokole	Adductor brevis femoris
Kapakahi	Pyriformis
Kaula lemu	Semitendinosus
Kau nui	Pectoralis major
Kau uuku	Pectoralis minor
Kikoo loihi	Peroneus longus
Kikoo pokole	Peroneus brevis
Kua uha	Vastus internus
Kuekue	Anconeus
Kuhi	Indicator
Kulana aoao maloko	Intercostales interni
Kulana aoao mawaho	Intercostales externi
Kumukolu	Triceps extensor cubiti
Kuoi	Pyramidalis
Kupono	Rectus abdominis
Lemu nui	Gluteus maximus
Lemu uuku	Gluteus minimus
Lemu waena	Gluteus medius
Libini	Plantaris
Maha	Temporalis
Mahoe	Gemini
Mimino	Levator labii superioris alaeque nasi
Mohala lima iki	Extensor minimi digiti
Mohala manamanalima	Extensor digitorum communis
Mole nui	Teres major
Mole uuku	Teres minor
Nau	Masseter
Nihomole lalo	Serratus posticus inferior
Nihomole mua	Serratus major anticus
Oakaloihi	Digastricus
Ohopelae	Occipito frontalis
Olapa ahalike	Pronator radii quadratus
Olapa iwi kano pokole	Supinator radii teres
Olapa kano loihi	Supinator radii longus
Olapa omole	Pronator radii teres
Ololi	Gracilis
Olona	Facialis or Tensor vaginae femoris
Olona lemu	Semimembranosus

Oloolo wawae maloko	Gastrocnemius internus or Soleus
Oloolo wawae mawaho	Gastrocnemius externus or Gemellus
Opa ihu	Constrictor nasi
Opeapea oloko	Pterygoides internus
Opeapea owaho	Pterygoides externus
Palahalaha kua	Latissimus dorsi
Pani oloko	Obturator internus
Pani owaho	Obturator externus
Papakole maloko	Iliacus internus
Pelu hope	Tibialis posticus
Pelu kumu manamanalima	Flexor digitorum sublimis
Pelu lehelehe lalo	Depressor labii inferioris
Pelu loihi o ka lima nui	Flexor longus pollicis
Pelu mua	Tibialis anticus
Pelu peahi oloko	Flexor carpi radialis
Pelu peahi owaho	Flexor carpi ulnaris
Pelu welau manamanalima	Flexor digitorum profundus vel perforans
Poailihilihi	Orbicularis palpebrarum
Poaiwaha	Orbicularis oris
Poholima	Palmaris longus
Pokole	Popliteus
Pololei malalo	Rectus inferior
Pololei maloko	Rectus internus
Pololei maluna	Rectus superior
Pololei mawaho	Rectus externus
Pololei uha	Cruralis or Cruraeus
Poolua	Biceps fluxor cruris
Puhi	Buccinator
Pukupuku kuemaka	Corrugator supercilii
Uala	Biceps flexor cubiti
Uhao nui	Psoas magnus
Uhao uuku	Psoas parvus
Uhau lua	Longissimus dorsi
Uhau mua	Sacro-lumbalis
Uluna	Brachialis internus
Umauma	Triangularis or Sterno-costales
Upoho	Subscapularis

GLOSSARY 3
ENGLISH–HAWAIIAN

abdomen	*kea hakahaka*
acid	*acida*
anterior fontanel	*manawa mua*
antrum	*ana*
anvil bone (ear)	*iwi kua*
ascending/inferior vena cava	*aakoko e pii ana*
astragalus	*iwi kuekue*
back bone	*iwi kua*
bicuspids	*kui*
bile	*au*
blood vessel,	*aa*
or vessel in general in the body	
bone	*iwi*
brain	*lolo*
bronchi	*manamana makalii*
buttocks bone	*iwi lemu*
calcaneum	*iwi ami*
calcium	*puna*
carpal bone	*iwi pulima*
cartilage	*pilali*
cathartic medicine	*laau naha*
chest	*kea paa*
chewing muscle	*io nau*
clavicle	*iwi lei*
coccyx	*iwi okole*
concave	*upoho*
convex	*opuupuu*
coronary artery	*aalele puuwai*
coronary vein	*aakoko puuwai*
coronel suture	*hoai manawa*
cuboides	*iwi ahalike*
cuneiforme bone (hand)	*iwi makia*
cuspids	*ole*
descending/superior vena cava	*aakoko e iho ana*

diaphragm	*ka paku mawaena o ka naau a me ke ake mama*
disease	*mai*
duodenum	*naau kapuwai*
ear base	*kumupepeiao*
ear bone	*iwi pepeiao*
ethmoid bone	*iwi kanana*
eyebrow	*kuemaka*
eye socket	*makalua*
fan-shaped bone	*iwi peahi*
fat	*momona*
femur	*iwi hilo*
fibula	*iwi pili*
firm	*maloeloe*
first or medial cuneiform bone (foot)	*iwi makia mua*
floating joint	*hookuina lewa*
fluid	*wai*
fontanel	*manawa*
frontal bone	*iwi lae*
hard	*oolea*
head in thigh bone	*huamoa*
hearing nerve	*aalolo lohe*
heart	*puuwai*
hinged joint	*hookuina ami*
hip bone	*iwi papakole*
humerus	*iwi uluna*
hyoid bone	*iwi alelo (elelo)*
incisors	*niho ai waiu*
intestine	*naau*
joint	*ami*
kidney	*puupaa*
lachrymal bone	*iwi waimaka*
lambdoidal suture	*hoai kala*
left auricle	*pepeiao hema*
left ventricle	*opu hema*
left carotid artery	*aalele oa hema*
left subclavian artery	*aalele iwilei hema*
lever	*une*
ligament	*olona*
liver	*ake, akepaa*
lumbar bone	*iwi puhaka*
lunare bone (hand)	*iwi mahina*
lymphatic	*aaomo*
magnum bone (hand)	*iwi nui*

malar bone	*iwi papalina*
mallet bone (ear)	*iwi hamare*
mandible	*iwi a lalo*
maxilla	*iwi a luna*
medicine	*lapaau*
metacarpal bone	*iwi peahi lima*
metatarsus	*iwi peahi wawae*
molars	*kuinui*
muscle	*io*
naviculare bone (foot)	*iwi ipukai*
naviculare bone (hand)	*iwi waapa*
nerve	*aalolo*
nose bone	*iwi ihu*
occipital bone	*iwi hope*
olfactory nerve	*aalolo honi*
optic nerve	*aalolo nana*
orbiculare bone (hand)	*iwi poepoe*
pain	*eha*
palate bone	*iwi kileo*
palpitation	*kapalili*
parietal bone	*iwi hua*
patella	*iwi kuapoi*
pelvis	*iwi ka, puhaka*
permanent teeth	*niho paa*
perspiration	*hou*
perspiration produced by the steam covering over a fire; the patient sits covered with a kapa over it	*puholoholo*
petrous part	*hapa oolea*
phalange, toe	*iwi manamana wawae*
phalange, finger	*iwi manamanalima*
polypus	*iokupu*
posterior fontanel	*manawa hope*
protuberance	*puupuu*
pubic bone	*iwi puukole*
pulmonary artery	*aalele ake mama*
pulmonary vein	*aakoko ake mama*
radius	*iwi kano*
ribs	*iwi aoao*
right auricle	*pepeiao akau*
right carotid artery	*aalele oa akau*
right subclavian artery	*aalele iwilei akau*
right ventricle	*opu akau*
round bone	*iwi poepoe*

sacrum	*iwi kikala*
sagittal suture	*hoai kaupaku*
salivary glands	*anoano*
scapula	*iwi hoehoe*
second or intermediate	*iwi makia lua*
cuneiforme bone (foot)	
sesamoid bone	*iwi anoano*
shoulder bone	*iwi poohiwi*
sphenoid bone	*iwi opeapea*
spinal nerve	*aalolo kuamoo*
spleen	*ake niau*
sprain	*okupe*
squamous part	*hapa unahi*
square	*huinaha*
stapes (ear)	*iwi keehi*
sternum	*iwi umauma*
stomach	*opu*
styloid process	*kui*
suture	*hoai*
syphilis	*pala*
tarsus	*iwi puupuuwawae*
tear duct	*luauhane*
temporal bone	*iwi maha*
temporal suture	*hoai maha*
tendon	*kaula*
third or lateral	*iwi makia kolu*
cuneiforme bone (foot)	
thorax	*houpo*
thumb	*manamana nui*
tibia	*iwi ku*
tough	*uwauwa*
trachea	*kani ai*
trapezius bone (hand)	*iwi ewaewa*
tricuspid valve	*pani huina kolu*
turbinated bone	*iwi owili*
ulna	*iwi kubita*
unciforme bone (hand)	*iwi lou*
urinary bladder	*koana mimi*
valves	*pani aapu*
vertebrae	*iwi kuamoo*
vomer	*iwi paku*
wisdom teeth	*niho oo*
womb	*puao*

GLOSSARY 4
MUSCLES:
LATIN–HAWAIIAN

Adductor brevis femoris	*Kahela pokole*
Adductor longus femoris	*Kahela loihi*
Adductor magnus femoris	*Kahela nui*
Anconeus	*Kuekue*
Biceps flexor cubiti	*Uala*
Biceps fluxor cruris	*Poolua*
Brachialis internus	*Uluna*
Buccinator	*Puhi*
Constrictor nasi	*Opa ihu*
Coraco brachialis	*Kahalua*
Corrugator supercilii	*Pukupuku kuemaka*
Cruralis or Cruraeus	*Pololei uha*
Deltoid	*Kaha*
Depressor anguli oris	*Haikaikanuku*
Depressor labii inferior	*Pelu lehelehe lalo*
Digastricus	*Oakaloihi*
Extensor carpi radialis brevior	*Hoalapokole*
Extensor carpi radialis longus	*Hoalaloihi*
Extensor carpi ulnaris	*Hooala peahi*
Extensor digitorum communis	*Mohala manamanalima*
Extensor minimi digiti	*Mohala lima iki*
Extensor ossis metacarpi pollicis manus	*Hooala lima nui*
Extensor primi internodii	*Hoopololei mua o ka lima nui*
Extensor secundi internodii	*Hoopololei lua o ka lima nui*
Facialis or Tensor vaginae femoris	*Olona*
Flexor carpi radialis	*Pelu peahi oloko*
Flexor carpi ulnaris	*Pelu peahi owaho*
Flexor digitorum profundis perforans	*Pelu welau manamanalima*

Flexor digitorum sublimis	*Pelu kumu manamanalima*
Flexor longus pollicis	*Pelu loihi o ka lima nui*
Gastrocnemius externus	*Oloolo wawae mawaho*
or Gemellus	
Gastrocnemius internus or Soleus	*Oloolo wawoe maloko*
Gemini	*Mahoe*
Gluteus maximus	*Lemu mui*
Gluteus minimus	*Lemu uuku*
Gracilis	*Ololi*
Iliacus internus	*Papakole maloko*
Indicator	*Kuhi*
Infra spinatus	*Hoehoelalo*
Intercostales externi	*Kulana aoao mawaho*
Intercostales interni	*Kulana aoao maloko*
Latissimus dorsi	*Palahalaha kua*
Levator angulis oris	*Hooewanuku mua*
Levator labii superioris	*Mimino*
alaeque nasi	
Levator labii superioris proprius	*Hoopinana lehelehe luna*
Levator palpebrae superioris	*Kaakaamaka*
Longissimus dorsi	*Uhau lua*
Masseter	*Nau*
Obliquus ascendens internus	*Hio maloko*
Obliquus descendens externus	*Hiomawaho*
Obliquus inferior	*Auwiolalo*
Obliquus superior or Trochlearis	*Auwioluna*
Obturator externus	*Paniowaho*
Obturator internus	*Panioloko*
Occipito frontalis	*Ohopelae*
Orbicularis oris	*Poaiwaha*
Orbicularis palpebrarum	*Poailihilihi*
Palmaris longus	*Poholima*
Pectinalis	*Hena*
Pectoralis major	*Kau nui*
Pectoralis minor	*Kau uuku*
Peroneus brevis	*Kikoo pokole*
Peroneus longus	*Kikoo loihi*
Plantaris	*Libini*
Platysma myoides	*Eeke*
Popliteus	*Pokole*
Pronator radii quadratus	*Olapa ahalike*
Pronator radii teres	*Olapa omole*
Psoas magnus	*Uhao nui*
Psoas parvus	*Uhao uuku*

Pterygoides externus	*Opeapea owaho*
Pterygoides internus	*Opeapea oloko*
Pyramidalis	*Kuoi*
Pyriformis	*Kapakahi*
Quadratus femoris	*Ahalike uha*
Quadratus luborum	*Ahalike puhaka*
Rectus abdominis	*Kupono*
Rectus externus	*Pololei mawaho*
Rectus femoris or Rectus cruris	*Alaea*
Rectus inferior	*Pololei malalo*
Rectus internus	*Pololei maloko*
Rectus superior	*Pololei maluna*
Rhomboides	*Huinaha hio kua*
Sacro-lumbalis	*Uhau mua*
Sartorius	*Hoahaaha*
Semimembranosus	*Olona lemu*
Semitendinosus	*Kaula lemu*
Serratus major anticus	*Nihomolemua*
Serratus posticus inferior	*Nihomole lalo*
Splenius	*Apana*
Sterno-cleido-mastoideus	*Alawa*
Subscapularis	*Upoho*
Supinator radii longus	*Olapa kano loihi*
Supinator radii teres	*Olapa iwi kano pokole*
Supraspinatus	*Hoehoeluna*
Temporalis	*Maha*
Teres major	*Mole nui*
Teres minor	*Mole uuku*
Tibialis anticus	*Pelu mua*
Tibialis posticus	*Pelu hope*
Transversalis abdominis	*Iliwai*
Trapezius or Cucullaris	*Hokua*
Triangularis or Sternocostales	*Umauma*
Triceps extensor cubiti	*Kumukolu*
Vastus Externus	*Alo uha*
Vastus Internus	*Kua uha*
Zygomaticus major	*Hooewanuku waena*
Zygomaticus minor	*Hooewanuku hope*

REFERENCES

Abraham, P. H., R. T. Hutchings, and S. C. Marks, Jr. *McMinn's Color Atlas of Human Anatomy*. 4th ed. London: Mosby, 1998.

Alexander, W. D. *A Brief History of the Hawaiian People*. Honolulu, 1891.

American Heritage Dictionary. Boston: Houghton Mifflin Co., 1971.

Andrews, Lorrin. *Vocabulary of the Hawaiian Language*. Lahaina: Lahainaluna Press, 1836.

———. *Dictionary of the Hawaiian Language*. Rutland, Vt. & Tokyo: Tuttle, 1974. Reprint, 1865 edition, H. M. Whitney, Honolulu.

Andrews, Robert W. "Lorrin Andrews and his Relation to Copperplate Engravings." *Friend* 72 (July 1906).

Brigham, W. *Ka Hana Kapa*. Honolulu: Bishop Museum Press, 1911.

Bushnell, O. A. "Hawaii's First Medical School." *Hawaii Historical Review* 2, no. 9 (October 1967).

Clark, E. W. "Mission Seminary, Lahainaluna, Maui." *Hawaiian Spectator*. V. 1. Honolulu, 1838.

Damon, Ethel M. *The Stone Church at Kawaiahao, 1820–1944*. Honolulu, 1945.

Dibble, Sheldon. *History of the Sandwich Islands*. Lahaina: Press of the Mission Seminary, 1843.

Dorland's Illustrated Medical Dictionary. Philadelphia: W. B. Saunders Co., 1985.

Feher, Joseph. *Hawaii: A Pictorial History*. Honolulu: Bishop Museum Press, 1969.

Fornander, Abraham. *An Account of the Polynesian Race*. V. 2. London, 1878–1885.

Fragments, II, IV, Family Record, House of Judd. Hawaiian Mission Children's Society Library, unpublished manuscripts.

Gardener, Ernest, Donald Gray, and Ronan O'Rahilly. *Anatomy*. 4th ed. Philadelphia: W. B. Saunders Co., 1975.

Gray, Henry. *Anatomy*. New York: Bounty Books, 1977.

Handy, E.S.C., and Elizabeth G. Haudy. *Native Planter in Old Hawaii.* Honolulu: Bishop Museum Press, 1972.

Hawaiian National Bibliography. V. 1. Compiler David W. Forbes. Honolulu: University of Hawai'i Press, 1999.

Judd, A. F. "On the Jubilee of the Hawaiian Bible." *Hawaiian Evangelical Association Reports, 1878–1889.* Honolulu, 1889.

Judd, G. P., IV. *Dr. Judd, Hawaii's Friend.* Honolulu: University of Hawai'i Press, 1960.

Judd, Laura. *Honolulu.* Chicago: Lakeside Press, 1966.

Kamakau, Samuel M. *Ruling Chiefs.* Honolulu: Kamehameha Schools, 1961.

Kuykendall, R. S. *The Hawaiian Kingdom.* V. 1. Honolulu: University of Hawai'i Press, 1968.

Lecker, George T. "Lahainaluna 1831–1877." M.A. thesis, University of Hawai'i, 1938.

Luquiens, H. M. "Engravings at Lahainaluna." *Friend* 103 (February 1933).

Missionary Album. Honolulu: Hawaiian Mission Children's Society, 1969.

Netter, Frank. *Atlas of the Human Anatomy.* East Hanover, N.J.: Novartis, 1989.

Nida, E. "Linguistics and Ethnology in Tranlation-Problems." *Word* 1, no. 2 (August 1945): 194–208.

Pukui, Mary K., and Samuel H. Elbert. *Hawaiian Dictionary.* Honolulu: University of Hawai'i Press, 1971.

Pukui, Mary K., E. S. Haertig, and C. A. Lee. *Nana i ke Kumu.* V. 1 Honolulu, 1972.

Rose, Roger G. *Hawaii the Royal Isles.* Honolulu: Bishop Museum Special Publication 67, 1980.

Smith, Jerome V. C. *The Class Book of Anatomy Designed for Schools.* 3rd ed. Boston: Robert S. David, 1837.

Strazer, Marie. *Na Paniolo o Hawaii.* Honolulu: State Foundation on Culture and the Arts, Academy of Arts, 1987.

van Patten, Nathan. "Early Native Engravers of Hawaii." *Papers of the Bibliographical Society of America* 20 (1926).

INDEX

abdomen, 51–55; muscles of, 70, 71

American Board of Commissioners for Foreign Missions, 1, 3, 5

Anatomia (Judd), xi–xiv, 1, 6; copper engravings in, xi, 2; early preparation of, x–xi, 3–4; print run, 5; publication of, 5

anatomy, 9

Andrews, Lorrin, 1, 2, 3–4

aorta, 45, 47, 48

arteries, 48–49; carotid, 47; subclavian, 48. *See also* aorta

back, muscles of, 73

Bailey, Edward, x

bile, 52

Blatchely, Abraham, 1

blood, 54–55; black, 43, 44, 46, 52; circulation of, 42–43, 46–47; red, 43, 46–47

bones of the human body, 10–11, 23–24; anus, 27; buttocks, 26; coccyx, 27; complete list of, 35–36; during childhood, 10, 12, 16; during pregnancy, 10; hip, 25–26; number of in the human body, 12; pelvis, 25–26; pubic, 26; ribs, 25; sacrum, 26–27; spine (vertebrae), 24–25; sternum, 25; types of, 11; use of fat in, 11. *See also other individually listed bones of the body*

brain, the, 37, 50

calcaneum, 33–34

calcium, 10–11, 55

cartilage, 10

chest, muscles of, 72

children, and digestion of solid food, 22

Clark, Ephraim, 2, 4

Class Book of Anatomy Designed for Schools (Smith), x, 3, 5

colon, the, 53

Cook, Captain, x

Cooke, Amos, 4

Dibble, Sheldon, 2

Dictionary of the Hawaiian Language (Andrews), 4

duodenum, 52, 53

ear, bones of, 14–15; back, 23; hammer, 23; round, 23; stirrup, 23

ear, muscles of, 41

eye sockets, 16, 19, 20

face, bones of, 18; cheek (malar), 19; hyoid, 22; lachrymal, 20; lower jaw, 21; nasal, 19; palate, 20; partition, 21; turbinated, 20; upper jaw, 19

floating joints, 28–29

189

ABOUT THE TRANSLATOR

Esther T. Mookini taught Hawaiian language at Kapiolani Community College, University of Hawai'i. Since her retirement, she has worked as a volunteer at the Hawaii Judiciary History Center, where she translates court documents. Together with Samuel H. Elbert and Mary Kawena Pukui, she is the author of *Place Names of Hawaii*, a primary Hawaiian studies resource book.